IMAGERY
OF
CANCER

IMAGERY OF

IMAG

An Evaluation Tool fc

INSTITUTE FOR PERSONALITY AND ABILITY TESTING
CHAMPAIGN, ILLINOIS

CANCER

⌐CA

e Process of Disease

Jeanne Achterberg/G. Frank Lawlis

With Foreword by Beatrix Cobb

Library of Congress Cataloging in Publication Data

Achterberg, Jeanne, 1942-
    Imagery of cancer (IMAGE-CA).

    Bibliography: p.
    Includes index.
    1. Cancer. 2. Mental healing. 3. Imagery
(Psychology) I. Lawlis, G. Frank, joint author.
II. Title. [DNLM: 1. Neoplasms--Psychology.
2. Imagination. QZ200 A179i]
RC271.M4A23   616.9'94'0019   77-90181
ISBN 0-918296-10-2

Institute for Personality and Ability Testing
1602 Coronado Drive, Champaign, Illinois

Printed in the United States of America.

Production Editor: Jay L. Sherman; Cover design by Zimmerman and Associates

DEDICATION

The IMAGE-CA was developed during a metamorphosis in our lives, and in some sense we must regard it as the creative product of that profound change. During the year that the data were collected, analyzed, and tentatively described for publication, we met, recognized our mutual archetypes, fell in love, and married. We would like to dedicate the book first and foremost to our eternal relationship.

We would like to also acknowledge the professional support that encouraged us to extend our abilities into the controversial area of cancer research: To Dr. Carl and Stephanie Simonton who allowed us access to patients and to their insights, to Bz Cobb whose training provided a firm foundation for the research, to Bob Butler who vocalized his belief in the direction that we were taking, and to Dr. Phala Helm and the Cancer Rehabilitation Project which provided us a rich opportunity for substantiating our intuitions.

Our appreciation for emotional support is expressed to our five children for their loving tolerance of professional parents, to Myrtle Thomas for her special care, to Karen Nyquist for far more than manuscript preparation, and to Marie Norris for her unusual wisdom. Our thanks to the variety of affiliations and resources that allowed the data to be collected and analyzed, despite the fact that funding for this area of research produces a monumental problem. The Institute of Noetic Science provided the Simontons with a grant that assisted partially with data collection, data analysis was defrayed through a grant from the North Texas State University, and the second normative study for the IMAGE-CA was subsumed under a patient evaluation effort funded by NCI Contract #N01-CN-45133.

Finally, and probably most important, we remain very indebted to the many patients who so graciously allowed us to conduct the study. If and when a universal holistic approach to cancer management is accepted, we have little doubt that it will largely be because of the kind of patient generosity in sharing personal and difficult insights such as we encountered through our research. We have attempted to treat their protocols with the respect, honor, and admiration that they deserve.

Jeanne Achterberg, Ph.D.
G. Frank Lawlis, Ph.D.

CONTENTS

FIGURES

TABLES

FOREWORD

For more than three decades, speculations concerning the impact and continuing role of psychological factors impinging upon the patient diagnosed as having cancer have intrigued medical and psychological members of the treatment team. These speculations, for the most part, have been subjective and intuitive, rather than clear-cut, demonstrable variables which could be reported objectively and considered, along with the physiological indices of the disease process, in the treatment plan. Perhaps the most relevant reason for this omission from the official medical history has been the fact that there was no standard, objective means of recording and evaluating these nebulous, but tantalizing clues to future course of the disease.

This book presents an exciting and well-documented instrument (IMAGE-CA) as a proposed answer to that dilemma! The IMAGE-CA was developed for the specific purpose of eliciting and interpreting applicable psychological elements with which most patients must cope while undergoing diagnostic and treatment process in cancer.

Achterberg and Lawlis, the authors, utilized a well-known concept in medicine, imagery, as the theoretic foundation in developing the protocol. The term "imagery" has a connotation of a subjective projective technique, but this is not the case with IMAGE-CA. With consummate skill and patience Achterberg and Lawlis have carefully formalized the imagery drawings and the ensuing inquiry interview procedures in such a way as to make possible objective scoring. Then, the administrative and scoring procedures have been painstakingly standardized to insure the possibility of across administrator and scorer integrity. Finally, two circumspect validation studies were accomplished. These studies found IMAGE-CA scores meaningful in both clinical interpretation and statistical prediction areas.

Both authors of this technique are highly competent and creative psychologists. They brought to this challenge the skills of an astute physiological psychologist and the judgment of a Diplomate in Counseling with a second specialization in statistical procedures. To this combined psychological expertise, the developers added consistent medical consultation, as well as individual participation as members of a medical-psychological team, in the evaluation and refinement of this instrument. Consequently, the protocol is germane to both medical and psychological research and clinical practice.

The authors do not offer this instrument as an accomplished end product. Rather, they see it as an important first step toward a goal of making possible scientific research in the psychophysiological understanding of the emotional components of the baffling disease known as cancer. They solicit continued study and utilization of the technique in an effort to refine and validate its worth.

It would seem that this technique could hold a pertinent three-fold value for those involved in the all-out war against cancer. First, it is a way to formalize the observations of the treatment team in such a way as to focus on the emotional trauma endured by the patient suffering from the disease, and as physician understanding of these psychological stresses increase, enhanced communication between doctor and patient should be apparent. Second, as a standardized instrument, which allows for statistical prediction as well as clinical interpretation, it should expedite accomplishment of psychophysiological research so pertinent to the study of this intricate disease entity. Finally, the very presence of such an instrument in the literature could act as a stimulus to challenge the creativity of other researchers, not only to test the effectiveness of this protocol, but to develop additional tools as well. Altogether, this work should lead to a more sophisticated approach to investigations focused upon the elucidation of elusive psychophysiological correlates and interactions in the long-standing medical riddle called cancer.

Beatrix Cobb, Ph.D.

Horn Professor in Psychology
Texas Tech University
Lubbock, Texas
August, 1977

I

INTRODUCTION

Like most terminal diseases, intimate contact with cancer spurs the scientist to discover its cause and cure. That being beyond the present realm of possibility, a reasonable understanding of the ways in which cancer patients deal with the disease in a constructive fashion can be pursued in order to aid in the medical treatment. As students of the body, we began to ask questions about the role patients play in their prognosis and treatment. Is the patient simply a mosaic of organs, and disease merely an obstacle to their functioning? Is it justifiable to view the physician or surgeon as a mechanic modifying or adapting the motor to regain functioning; whereas, the patient is passive (and helpless) to both the doctor and disease?

From a broad and extensive review of the literature, we found abundant evidence to suggest that both quality and quantity of life measures were predicted by psychological dimensions, even to the extent of formulating hypotheses regarding premorbid variance and remediation in cancer. Rather than becoming entangled in a web of conjecture of impossible methodologies, we set out to determine what the patients themselves could tell us about their own understanding of what was happening to them and then to determine the accuracy of their prognoses. We formulated two specific goals in the research plan: (1) to understand the cancer patient from a holistic perspective to the extent that we could explain not only his behaviors in general, but how he behaved toward his diseases as well, and (2) to formalize this understanding in order to enable other health professionals to reach the most effective level of communication with the cancer patient.

Our first task was to find out what "language" to use in communicating with the patients and their disease. We found that through a relaxation exercise they could focus and imagine aspects of their disease. By instructing them to draw these images, and through a structured interview, we began to recognize 14 scorable dimensions for standardization and quantification. These were vividness, activity, and strength of the cancer cell, vividness and activity of the white blood cell, relative comparison of size and numbers of cancer and white blood cells, strength of white blood cell, vividness and effectiveness of medical treatment, degree of symbolism, overall strength of imagery, regularity of imagery process, and clinical opinion related to prognosis based on combined imagery factors.

The instrument itself was developed after several hundred hours of patient sessions—listening and questioning them on the manner in which they perceived their disease, immunity, and treatment. Over the course of time, the 14 dimensions stood out remarkably well as key aspects in the disease imagery. Our intuitions regarding the relationship between the dimensions and the disease were verified when we were able to relate the scores to follow-up criteria.

The first group of patients that we studied provided incredibly valuable insights. They were all well educated, highly verbal, and for the most part intimately familiar with relaxation, meditation, and imagery techniques. Many were physicians, psychologists, biologists, and in allied health fields, so that their own professional backgrounds enhanced their discussion beautifully. To them we owe a significant debt of gratitude, and an acknowledgment that they are truly educators in the disease process.

Our concern that the relationship between imagery and disease course might have been unique only to an elite group of psychologically oriented patients was dispelled when we applied the IMAGE-CA to county hospital patients, most of whom were indigent, poorly educated, and scarcely familiar with such things as the phagocytic activity of the white blood cells. When this latter group was instructed to become physically relaxed and quiet, and to take an imaginary trip through their bodies, their perceptions proved to be valid

4

prognosticators. These findings should serve to elevate cancer patients to new positions of personal responsibility and authority in disease management.

Fifty-eight cancer patients were used in the first validation study (Normative Group I) with disease status serving as a criterion. The predictive validity as well as concurrent validity of the instrument was upheld. A group of 22 lower class patients (Normative Group II) was the focus of the second effort. With this more homogeneous sample, functionability of the patients was the criterion. Both studies were consistent in reliability analyses and agreement checks. In both cases psychological and neurophysiological measures were correlated with the 14 dimensions in order to understand their relationships to other approaches. In a separate study with the technique (Achterberg, Lawlis, Simonton, & Simonton, 1977), it was found that psychological measures, especially the imagery dimensions, predicted disease progress much more accurately than blood chemistries.

Through our studies with the imagery technique and cancer patients, we feel that we have personally reached our first goal: to understand the cancer patient in a broader perspective. We can now predict from a variety of measurements the patients' expectancies and attitudes toward disease and treatment factors. We can more clearly understand the struggle for life. However, our goals also included helping others understand the cancer patients in confrontation with this dread disease. Consequently, we have attempted to formulate a specific approach designed to acquaint health professionals with methods that foster an understanding of patients and the role patients play in their own treatment. This book offers a systematic means of inviting patients' perceptions for hypothesis testing, in the same sense that physical data from the patients are obtained.

IMAGERY: A FOUNDATION FOR BEHAVIORAL MEDICINE

The notion of mental imagery, visualization, seeing with the mind's eye, or inner vision (or whatever one chooses

5

to call the introspective process that is accompanied by visual images) has an extraordinarily rich history in both psychology and medicine. In fact, it formed the basis for study in the first psychological laboratory established by Wundt in 1879. The scientific analysis of the content of the mind seemed to be an appropriate area of research for the fledgling discipline, and psychologists began to try to objectify the nebulous arena of the imagination. Because the early results were neither pragmatic nor interpretable, psychologists turned to the analysis of behavior as their focus, dismissing the more phenomenological aspects once again as grist for the theologians and philosophers.

At the same time that experimentalists were turning their attentions elsewhere, psychologists engaged in therapy were discovering and refining the various facets of imagery as a treatment modality. Imagery, after all, is the stuff that dreams are made of: it is a facilitator of memory, an integral part of creativity, and may well be a prerequisite for attitude change. The recapturing of mental images, a process which allows a patient to work through long-repressed conflict, lies at the heart of traditional Freudian analysis. Jung, too, believed that the trip through the unconscious via visualization techniques produced a wealth of insight, offering the patient a means of dealing more effectively with life situations. He also held that this procedure was capable of enhancing emotional growth and of leading to an understanding of the more ethereal, mystical qualities of human existence.

Uncountable new modes of psychotherapy rely heavily or exclusively on the manipulation of the visualization procedure. To refer to them as new, however, is somewhat misleading, since they are largely innovations based on methods that can be traced to early Egyptians, to Shaman rituals from many cultures, and to classical hypnosis as well. These schools of therapy include Psychosynthesis, Gestalt, and Arica, to mention but a few, and generally involve the achievement of some relaxed or altered state of consciousness, followed by suggestions of either concrete images or of spontaneous imagery with the purpose varying from attitude change to physiologic alteration. Regardless of the procedure,

6

the message is essentially the same: Image the type of person you wish to become, both in terms of mental and physiological factors, and through that process you will be more likely to reach your goals.

Scientific Analysis of Imagery

The renewed study of inner processes was recognized in 1964 by Robert Holt in an article in the *American Psychologist* entitled, "Imagery: The Return of the Ostracized." Imagery or visualization was welcomed back as an important area of scientific pursuit. Ironically, creative imagery has crept back into scientific psychology through a recognition of the basis for biofeedback procedures and counter-conditioning, both being practical applications of traditional learning theory. In the case of biofeedback, patients usually report some form of mental imagery that accompanies a change in autonomic function. Counter-conditioning stresses practice in visualizing a feared or noxious stimulus while in a relaxed physiological state. This latter therapy, particularly, acknowledges the delicate interplay between psyche and soma that is encouraged by the visualization technique.

In another context, Luria (1968) writing on eidectic imagery, has provided valuable information on the role of imagery in the learning-memory process. He and others have found that eidetic (or photographic) memory is not only an underlying phenomena of the learning process, but tends to diminish with age. Evidently the process of visual imagery or the storage of visual memories is in part replaced by verbal memory storage. We can probably safely assume that the ability to form visual images is normally distributed in the population and therefore does not remain the province of the few who exhibit pronounced photographic memory.

Neisser (1972), in discussing the difference between visualization and perception, claimed that the same kind of synthesis is involved in both, but in the case of visualization it is based on stored rather than on current incoming information. This view suggests that with the exception of the external input, the process of imagery involves the neurological substrates integral to the visual process itself.

7

The ability to form visual images has been examined by several investigators and found to correlate with psychological traits and abilities. Among those traits where a positive correlation exists are hypnotic susceptibility (Palmer & Field, 1968; Wagman & Stewart, 1974), ease of verbal learning (Paivio, 1969), personality characteristics of introversion/extraversion (Huckabee, 1974), confusion in consciousness (Richardson, 1969; Sheehan, 1973), and creative self-perceptions (Khatina, 1975).

Despite widespread interest, the measurement of the imagery experience, per se, remains a complex impediment to the understanding of the process since it consists of intrinsically private events which have remained externally unverifiable. Such complications are not new to psychology, however, since the "core" areas of the discipline such as learning, motivation, and perception have also been fraught with all the problems of the verification of hypothetical constructs.

While the ability to image and vividness of imagery have been fairly well studied in regard to relationships with certain events, the actual content of the imagery seems to have been neglected from an analytical viewpoint except in clinical report (e.g., Cautela, 1975). Yet the imagery content would seem to be most necessarily correlated with the outcome of the procedure. It is not merely the capability of the individual to image, but the nature of the image itself that eventuates in any change in attitude, perceptual, or physiological function.

Physiological Correlates of Imagery

Several studies have demonstrated that when the appropriate neuronal pathways are artificially stimulated by some means, images are experienced. For example, neither during dream sleep, nor during hallucinations, nor when visual pathways of the brain are electrically stimulated is the retina actually involved. We are forced to conclude that the fine line between external and internal visual reality is simply a matter of peripheral vs. no-peripheral stimulation. Images are "real" to the person experiencing them, and presumably because they share common neurological pathways with the externally produced images, they are capable of evoking the same physiological or psychological response.

Jacobsen's work (1942) has had a pronounced effect on our understanding of the physiological ramifications of mental imagery. His research indicated that during imagery there is measurable tension in the part of the body involved in the visualization. For example, there is tension in the muscles of the eye during visual imagery, in the muscles of speech during sub-vocal thought, and in leg muscles when one imagines running. This tension merely reflects the involvement of conscious control over voluntary muscle groups and is, therefore, certainly no mystery. However, this consequence of mental imagery has led writers to propose advantages to mentally imaging or rehearsing physical feats prior to their exhibition (tennis players, golfers, and basketball players as well as others have professed to using some form of imagery).

Luria (1968) has also described the relationship of mental imagery to physiological response. He reported on a most unusual patient, adept at eidetic imagery, who was able to increase his heart rate significantly by imagining himself running to catch a train, and could decrease his heart rate back to normal by imaging himself in bed trying to go to sleep. In another experiment the subject was able to differentially raise the temperature of one hand by imaging his hand on a hot stove; again to decrease the temperature by seeing himself squeeze a piece of ice. His amazing subject was also able to alter pupil size by visualizing light, and could likewise influence the cochlear reflex by imaging a sudden sound. Admittedly, Luria was working with an exceptional patient, but as is the case with most advances, we learn by studying the anomalies.

The physiological effects of the mental imagery process has been documented by Drs. Schultz and Luthe (1969) in their compilation of 2400 studies based on the use of autogenic therapy. This therapeutic technique involves the use of visualization and relaxation procedures, offered in a highly structured framework. Changes accompanying the procedures often include alterations in temperature, blood sugar, blood pressure, white blood cell count, and brain wave

9

patterns. However, many of these changes occur naturally by relaxation alone. Therefore the relationship between visualization and relaxation and the relative contribution of each to the end result is still unclear.

The achievement of physical relaxation seems to greatly enhance the production of visual images (Richardson, 1969). Therefore, in a therapeutic context, relaxation techniques usually serve as a prelude to imagery suggestions. Total relaxation seems to be required in order for a patient to focus internally, to obliterate the demands made on the central nervous system by the maintenance and experience of muscular tension, and to gate out diversionary external stimuli. The ability to achieve a relaxed state also involves imagery to some extent, however. The patient usually imagines tension in some way flowing out of the body; he sees muscles changing in their form and state; the body warming via some internal production of heat. On another level, Benson (1975) and his colleagues have identified a series of physiological responses associated with simple relaxation. These responses can be thought of as conducive to a reestablishment of the body's equilibrium or homeostasis. They include lowered blood pressures, increased blood flow, decreased heart rate, intensification of alpha response, and a general decrease in metabolic processes indicated by decreased oxygen consumption and carbon dioxide production as well as a decrease in respiration. Benson calls the conglomerate response a wakeful, hypometabolic state which indicates the organism is mentally alert, but physically exhibits decreased sympathetic nervous system activity.

Imagery in Medicine

In view of the wide range of physical events that have been correlated with the production of visual imagery, a relationship between images and the healing or disease process logically follows. The use of visualization to promote healing may well have been the first form of the practice of medicine, and may also influence the effectiveness of any medical procedure. It stands to reason that in antiquity imagery would have been used to combat disease. Sickness,

like any other unexplained event, was attributed to malevo-
lent, unseen spirits. Quite logically, thought forms were then
used to combat thought forms. Historical records from Baby-
lonia, Assyria, Summaria, and Greece describe elaborate
rituals for ridding the body of disease. Most of these ancient
cultures relied on a practitioner skilled in the arts of visualization to guide the afflicted person through various thoughts,
dreams, or appeals to the gods to effect a healing. Many of
these same procedures are currently being practiced by
Indian tribes, particularly the Navaho and Canadian Eskimo
tribes. Trance-inducing ceremonies which are intended to
assist the Shaman with diagnostic insight are performed, after
which he applies the tools of his trade (herbs, sand painting,
lay on of hands, and a heavy dose of hypnotic suggestion). (We
heartily recommend Samuels & Samuels' *Seeing with the
Mind's Eye*, 1975, for a graphic presentation of these and
other imagery materials).

It has only been a recent development that medicine
or healing is considered a separate discipline. For centuries, it
was a free-for-all, with contributory statements made by
virtually every philosophical and religious group concerned
with the nature of man. Interestingly, the use of imagery as a
tool for retaining or regaining health is found in Christian
doctrine, Buddhism, Hinduism, in the Kaballist tradition of
Judaism, Hermetic and Palatonic philosophy, and in Rosicru-
cianism. In all of these, the functions of the mind have
supremacy over the physical attributes which are believed to
be only the concretion or manifestation of the former.

During the last century there have been a handful of
physicians who, perhaps as a response to frustration over the
variance in effectiveness of pills and surgery, developed alternative methods of healing based on imagery. Drs. Herbert
Benson, J. H. Schultz, Irving Oyle, Mike Samuels, Grantly
Dick-Read, and Carl Simonton are only a few of those physicians who have pioneered nontraditional techniques in a
variety of medical practices from obstetrics to oncology. Their
work has been enhanced and supported by experimental
psychologists and personality theorists who have illuminated
psychological correlates of various diseases and elucidated
involvement of the central nervous system in psychophysio-
logic disorder.

11

Probably the most extensive development of visualization as an adjunctive medical treatment is the autogenic therapeutic procedures developed by Schultz in the 1930s. Luthe (1969) reports on a complicated series of the Schultz exercises in which the patient is advised to visualize the heaviness in extremities, to imagine a peaceful scene, to concentrate on a feeling of warmth, to attain "mental contact" with vital organs, and to become involved in deep breathing. Specific visualizations include spontaneously imaged colors, objects, concepts, feelings, and questions asked of one's inner self. Schultz and Luthe describe prescriptions of particular visualizations to treat virtually every category of diseases including ulcers, gall bladder, colitis, heart condition, obesity, diabetes, *ad infinitum.*

A more specific use of imagery in medicine was designed for cancer patients by Dr. O. Carl Simonton, a radiation oncologist, and Stephanie Matthews-Simonton, a cancer counselor. Their practice, frequently termed one of the most innovative trends in medicine, combines both Eastern and Western approaches to health care. A description of the philosophy underlying the development of their treatment methods and their early approaches is provided by the Simontons in the *Journal of Transpersonal Psychology* (1975). A more recent overview is given in *Mind as Healer, Mind as Slayer* (Pelletier, 1977). The therapy itself is a collage of techniques, with an overriding acknowledgment and incorporation of the research on psychosocial aspects of the disease. A primary emphasis is on regular relaxation and guided imagery.

Anyone who attempts to cross disciplinary lines is likely to be severely criticized. Established paradigms are threatened by innovative ideas and new ways of looking at old issues. Medicine is particularly cautious—usually with great justification—and the Simontons are especially vulnerable. However, from our vantage point and having worked closely with their patients, negative criticism of their work is largely undeserved and is primarily based on incomplete information.

The IMAGE-CA was spawned after 20 months of testing, interviewing, researching their patients, and observing the Simontons practice their healing art. The patients had a remarkable story to tell involving very intensive detail of their cancer imagery and their ability to overcome the disease via a combination of internal mechanisms and medical treatment. As psychologists accustomed to being respectful of mental phenomena, this was not a surprise, and as researchers we were intrigued by the Simontons' use of imagery in treatment of the disease.

Our belief is that the Simontons, like other sensitive and experienced professionals, soon develop "internal correlations" in their heads. They learn "what leads to what," often incorporating a host of subtle and nonverbal cues. But, if the correlations can be demonstrated as reliable sources of prediction, then that person can be termed an artist. And if these correlations can be taught effectively to other people, then these correlations become a technology in their own right, available for more exploration and perfection, perhaps even to become a significant breakthrough in understanding.

We maintain that every physician utilizes some form of imagery in communicating with patients; that it is the process involved in building a "will to live"; that it is the expectation transmitted to the patient regarding the ability to return to health. In addition, it may be an underlying factor in the "bedside" manner of the physician which conveys, among other things, an expectancy to the patient involving the medical expertise. We also maintain that the placebo effect, or what the patient imagines (or images) "ought" to happen following medical administration directly guides disease progress, and is inseparable from medical practice.

Despite the fact that visualization has been an important part of healing throughout history, that it constitutes the basis for a new movement in medicine, and that it, albeit unsystematically, is involved in all forms of patient/physician interaction, it was not well studied in terms of its relationship to subsequent disease process prior to the development of the IMAGE-CA. The implications from the use of the instrument are many. For example, if an individual is able to visualize the internal condition of his or her body, we might imply that patients themselves can be superb diagnosticians. If various visualizations consistently relate to subsequent bodily processes, we might suggest the patient is also capable of

13

prognostication. At the extreme end, imagerial ability implies not only foresight but the ability to alter the disease course itself.

This viewpoint elevates the patient to new roles, and a new responsibility is placed with us in maintaining and becoming aware of and in tune with our bodies. Are patients simply capable of reflecting what is going on in their bodies and of predicting what will transpire as a result of being helpless victims of psychophysiological onslaught, or do they have a measure of control? This latter question has not been answered and requires conscious measurement and manipulation of the imagery procedure.

A Psychophysiological Model of Cancer Imagery

The theoretical basis for the relationship between physical disease and the cognitive processes reflected in a patient's imagery are derived from three factors: (1) the surveillance theory of cancer development; (2) the distress associated with the development of disease; and (3) principles of biofeedback (Achterberg, Simonton, & Matthews-Simonton, 1976). According to the surveillance theory (Prehn, 1969), abnormal cells occur occasionally within an organism but are usually successfully attacked by the body's immune system which is a combination of factors primarily involving the white blood cells. Only rarely does this system break down and allow clinical malignancy to develop. The cancer cells, rather than being strong, are viewed as metabolically confused and vulnerable to the normal attacking properties of the white blood cells. Secondly, the literature on the relationship between stress and cancer as well as other diseases is quite conclusive: both psychological and physiological stress can lead to a breakdown in host resistance through alterations in hormonal levels and in related dysfunctions of the immune system components (Riley, 1975; Solomon & Amkraut, 1972). Finally, the work on biofeedback has led to an awareness of the ability to consciously control body functions that were previously thought of as autonomic. Heart rate, blood flow, gastric processes, temperature, and other functions have been shown in innumerable studies to be conditionable, with the

14

crucial factor being the ability of the patient to monitor or observe these functions. So, taken together, these three factors strongly suggest that psychological processes can interact with natural physical processes in the development of disease, and that, conversely, a patient can use these factors to gain control of physiological functioning.

The proposed mechanism for the interaction between psychological and physical factors is diagrammed in Figures 1 and 2. The model is derived principally from the work of Hans Selye (1956) and involves much of what is known about the physiological concomitants of stress. The emotions accompanying stress—fear, anxiety, and depression—are reflected in limbic system activity, which directly involves hypothalamic and pituitary function. The pituitary, the body's master gland, regulates all hormonal activity. Furthermore, imbalances in hormonal activity have frequently been demonstrated to be connected to increases in malignant growth. Oversecretion of the adrenal has been particularly noted to affect the thymus and lymph integrity and subsequently the white blood cells. Stress can thus be viewed as having a twofold influence on the malignant process: (1) the production of abnormal cells increases, and (2) the capability of the body to destroy these cells is diminished. Imagery moving in a positive direction may serve to alleviate the disruptive emotional condition and thereby intervene in the stress—disease—stress cycle.

Psychophysiological Aspects of Cancer: Historical Perspectives

Decades of medical research have yielded no significant breakthroughs on cancer etiology. Although correlational findings continue to accumulate, we are far from understanding the fundamental cause as well as the mysterious course of the disease. Failure to adequately investigate the relevance of psychological variables may be the reason for the current impasse. It is generally accepted that many human disorders such as allergies, bronchial asthma, coronary artery disease, diabetes mellitus, epilepsy, hypertension, migraine, neurodermatitis, obesity, rheumatoid arthritis, and ulcerative

Figure 1

PSYCHOPHYSIOLOGICAL MODEL OF CANCER GROWTH

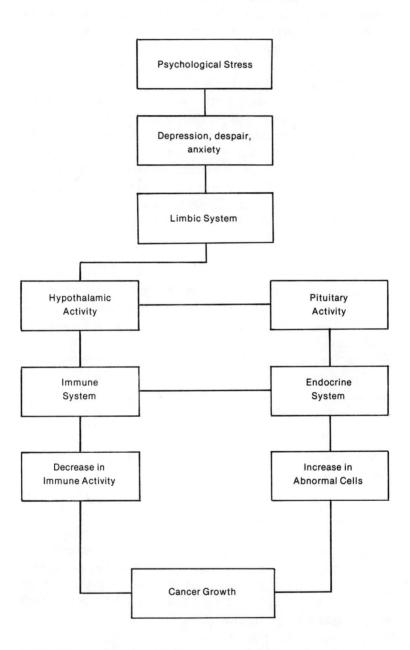

Figure 2

PSYCHOPHYSIOLOGICAL MODEL OF CANCER REGRESSION

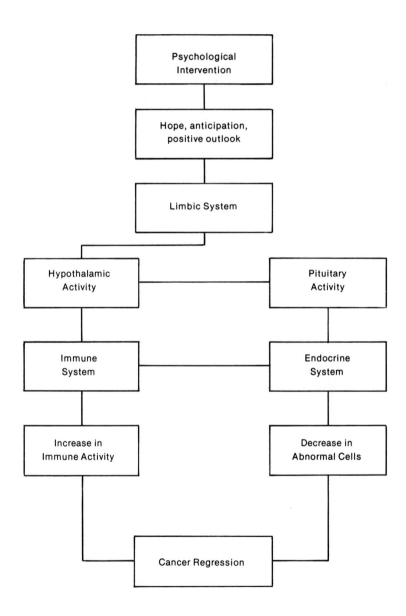

colitis have significant psychogenic aspects. Thus, it is not unreasonable to presume that a psychophysiological approach to the study of cancer may produce significant results.

The impression given by cancer research is that investigators, in general, have been trying to substantiate hypotheses which form part of an outmoded theory of specific cellular disease. Such a concept has become less and less tenable. Human behavior cannot be based solely on the laws of individual cell action. The functioning of individual cells is the result, and not necessarily the origin, of organized living. Cancer is no more a disease of cells than a traffic jam is a disease of cars. A lifetime study of the internal combustion engine would not help anyone to understand traffic problems.

The dilemma of cancer research is further exemplified by the increasing obscurity of much of the writing, the extraordinary remoteness, range, and intricacy of the papers presented, and by their failure to clarify the problem. Information accumulates rapidly while understanding lags far behind. What remains very clear, however, is that the incidence of cancer for most sites is steadily increasing, and that deaths from the disease have not decreased despite some prolongation of life following diagnosis.

A parallel may be drawn between the pre-Freudian attitude toward mental illness and the present day attitude toward cancer. Not until the 20th century did psychologists realize that mental disorder is related to the life experiences, life patterns, and personality configurations of those afflicted. Previously, mental illness, for all practical purposes, had been thought to result from the intrusion of some external agent, be it an "evil spirit," a microbe, or a chemical substance. At best the consensus was, and occasionally still is, that the mental patient was the arbitrary victim of an unknown and unexplained disease process within his brain. This general attitude toward mental aberrations prevailed until Charcot, Breuer, and Freud uncovered the extensive psychological patterns related to the neurotic symptoms of their patients. These findings revolutionized both diagnostic rrocedures and treatment methods of mental disorders and ushered in the general dynamic approach to the understanding of mental disorder.

18

Curiously, a similar development did not occur in medicine. Although deterministic and developmental theories were formulated early in biology (Lamarck, 1830; Darwin, 1901), the medical sciences as yet have not absorbed and integrated these realistic, holistic, and encompassing approaches to disease but instead have perpetuated what might be called a modified "witchcraft concept" of disease. From a medical point of view, most somatic illnesses are still understood to result from an invasion from without. Because the responsible agent is believed to exist outside and independent of the patient, most somatic diseases are still conceived of as striking individuals in an arbitrary and random fashion rather than expressing a condition determined and produced by the total organism set within the frame of its biological past, present, and its total environment. The patient is viewed as a hapless victim of these circumstances. Although medical research (e.g., Hinkle, Christenson, Benjamin, & Wolf, 1962) has shown empirically that even infectious diseases appear more often in anxious and depressed individuals rather than varying only with the degree of exposure to the bacteria, the general medical view has remained that somatic illness is an unpredictable condition which randomly may afflict anyone, and that somehow the cause is external to and independent of the individual (Bahnson & Bahnson, 1964a). The psychosomatic approach to cancer has been developed in reaction to such a mystically based and naive view of illness.

Cancer and Psychological Processes

In preparing this section we have reviewed nearly 50 studies, dating back to 1839, which have examined the relationship between psychological processes and cancer. Rather than describing each of these studies, a summary of the instrumentation and psychological variables found to relate to malignancy is presented in Table 1.

There are two general conclusions that are evident from this research. First, regardless of instrumentation, there are enough replications to formalize the notion that a relationship does exist between the course of the disease and psychological dimensions. Second, several premorbid psychological

19

Table 1

LITERATURE SUMMARY OF PSYCHOLOGICAL FACTORS RELATED TO CANCER

Author(s)	Year	Instrumentation	N	Psychological Factors Related to Cancer
Walshe	(1846)	observation	unknown	"woman of high color and sanguinous temperament"
Paget	(1870)	observation	unknown	deep anxiety, deferred hope and disappointment
Snow	(1883, 1890, 1893)	observation	250	depression
Evans	(1926)	psychotherapy progress	100	the last of a major catharsis
Foque	(1931)	observation	unknown	sad emotions
Miller & Jones	(1948)	observation	6	frequent occurrence of emotional difficulties
Bacon, Renneker, & Cutler	(1952)	case history	40	masochistic character inhibited sexuality and motherhood, inability to discharge anger
Greene	(1954, 1966)	interview	20	loss of significant other
Jacobs	(1954)	observation	unknown	self-destructiveness
Greene, Young, & Swisher	(1956)	observation	32	unresolved attachment to mother
Inman	(1964)	case study	1	guilt over masturbation
Muslin, Gyarfas, & Pieper	(1966)	questionnaires	74	separation from significant other
Greene	(1966)	observation	100	sadness, anxiety, anger, or hopelessness
Paloucek & Graham	(1966)	observation	88	psychosocial trauma and poor childhood
Kissen	(1967)	interview	930	disturbed relationships in childhood, ongoing adverse life situations
Blumberg	(1954)	MMPI, Rorschach	50	defensiveness, anxiety, low ability to reduce tension
Ellis & Blumberg	(1954)	case studies		low ability to reduce tension

Author	Year	Method	N	Findings
Bugental	(1954)	MMPI (Blumberg's sample)		brooding, useless, lacking in energy
Wheeler & Caldwell	(1955)	Rorschach	60	labile, preoccupation with sexual body, inhibited with early sex experiences, close attachment with mother
LeShan & Worthington	(1956)	Worthington Personal History	152	loss of important relationship, inability to express hostility, anxiety over death
Kissen & Eysenck	(1962)	Maudsley Personal Inventory	116	extraversion, neuroticism
Coppen & Metcalfe	(1964)	Maudsley Personal Inventory	47	extraversion
Nemeth & Mezei	(1954)	Rorschach	50	few M, lower 4%, passive hostility
Booth	(1964)	Rorschach	93	rigid guilt feelings toward others
Evans, Stern, & Marmorston	(1965)	adjective checklist	56	submissiveness
Netzer	(1965)	Taylor Manifest Anxiety Scale Neuroticism Scale, DAP	50	body image distortions, denial, fear of loss of control, neuroticism
Kissen	(1966)	interview, MMPI	150	incidences of child behavior problems
Koenig, Levin, & Brennan	(1967)	MMPI	36	depression
Tarlau & Smalheiser	(1951)	interview, Rorschach, DAP	11	mother-child relationship
Cobb	(1952)	Rorschach, interview	100	anticipatory fears and under-lying dependency
Reznikoff	(1955)	TAT, sentence completion	50	birth order and family domesticity, sadness, negative feelings
Bahnson & Bahnson	(1964b)	Rorschach	12	superficial extraversion, low empathy, "flattened" affect, rigid, constricted
LeShan	(1966)	Worthington Research Life History	450	early childhood relationship problems, recent adult event, loneliness
Bahnson & Bahnson	(1966)	interview	49	denial and repression of impulses
Achterberg & Lawlis	(1978)	Image-Ca, MMPI, Firo-B		denial, imagery, negative self-investment
Thomas	(1976)	questionnaire		early neglect

factors consistently appear. For example, the memory of an early home life inadequate to needs of support and security, a pre-disease event of an emotional loss, and feelings described as helplessness or hopelessness all emerged in several independent investigations.

Although many of the studies utilized standardized psychological measurement, the instruments used were primarily developed for diagnosis of mental illness. Therefore, the conceptualizations involved may be inadequate or inappropriate when applied to seriously ill patients, particularly if used to determine psychotherapeutic interventions. For this reason as well as others, the impact of psychological findings on the medical community has been slight. The jargon in psychological testing (such as "extraversion," "archetypes,") does little to facilitate interdisciplinary communication.

The heavy emphasis in the literature on attempting to define a cancer personality based on retrospective (post-diagnosis) information has not yielded much practical information for the health practitioner. In the first place, data gathered in this manner is of questionable validity; and secondly, premorbid psychological dimensions and events are not specific to present or future perspectives. There is very little one can do about past history or events that occur as a consequence of time. Clearly, in order to develop a better understanding of disease management, practitioners need new instrumentation specific to cancer and its psychological components. Therefore, the objectives for the design and construction of the IMAGE-CA were as follows:

1. *The instrument should form a closer communication link between physician and patient.* As medical training is intensified from year to year with more and more information available, the physician's learning becomes focused on the pathologies of organs and specific diagnosis, rather than on getting to know the patients. As the need for specialists grows, the patient becomes more a mosaic for referral sources than a personality.

This description is not intended as a criticism of medical training. There are logical reasons for these developments, such as the tremendous volume of medical information to learn and high caseloads. However, these factors have also placed the patient in a position of passivity; left behind in understanding and terminology.

2. *The instrument should assist the patient to participate in the rehabilitation process.* As a natural consequence of good communication with one's physician, the patient can more effectively aid his own remediation. As any physician will admit, medication or surgery can only assist the body in the natural process. If the patient understands the intent of the medical treatment, two things tend to happen. He or she gains hope and self-confidence, and trust in the physician. The resultant positive attitude often contributes as much to health as anything else. There are numerous case studies which have demonstrated healthy responses once patients have gained the anticipatory reaction associated with hope.

Through research in biofeedback we know that people have the capacity to control a variety of bodily responses, provided a monitoring device is available. Moreover, research has shown that subjects can demonstrate autonomic control with selected imagery as well as, if not better than, with a bio-feedback apparatus system.

Why couldn't patients be educated as to what autonomic systems need to be energized or slowed down, and be encouraged to image their recovery? Through control of thought processes a state of mind conducive to remediation could be developed at the very least, with the potential of significant healing at best.

3. *The instrument should allow the physician to anticipate the course of disease.* As affirmed by the research results, the course of cancer and probably other disease groups as well can be better predicted by psychological variables than medical measures (Achterberg, et al., 1977). This prediction is not surprising due to the fact that blood chemistries, blood pressure, and other physical measures are primarily reactive to disease state. Therefore, the physician using these measures is always predicting from a post hoc dimension. With the development of predictive measurement, the physician can provide treatment protocols for future disease

23

complications as well as engaging psychological intervention methods, if needed.

II

IMAGE-CA

The Technique

The Imagery technique utilizes two media of communication which are of mutual importance: (1) a personalized drawing of the disease components, and (2) a structured interview. Specifically, the approach is to guide the patient through relaxation exercises and then through a focus on the disease process. There is a subtle educational process during which the patient is instructed to imagine the cancer cells, the immunological system represented by white blood cells, and any medical treatment in whatever way he wishes. After the patient is given the opportunity to actively image this process, he is asked to draw his thoughts for the examiner. The interview is an attempt to clarify and objectify the meanings underlying the patient's drawings. The drawings and interview are then scores on the following 14 dimensions using 5-point scales:

1. Vividness of the cancer cell.
2. Activity of the cancer cell.
3. Strength of the cancer cell.
4. Vividness of the white blood cell.
5. Activity of the white blood cell.
6. Relative comparison of numbers of cancer cells to white blood cells.
7. Relative comparison of the size of cancer cells to white blood cells.
8. Strength of the white blood cell.
9. Vividness of the medical treatment (radiation, chemotherapy, surgery, etc.).

10. Effectiveness of the medical treatment.
11. Concreteness vs. symbolism.
12. Overall strength of imagery; emotional investment the patient projects to his drawing.
13. Estimated regularity of the number of times per day the patient thinks of his disease in the described way.
14. A clinical opinion by the examiner as to the prognosis for disease.

The 14 scale scores are then weighted and summed, yielding an overall Imagery Score. A more complete and detailed description of administration and scoring procedures follows.

ADMINISTRATION OF THE IMAGE-CA

Information on which judgments are based for the IMAGE-CA consists of:

1. Drawings of (a) the cancer cell, or the disease
   - (b) the immune system (usually referred to as white blood cells)
   - (c) any treatment for the malignancy

   and

2. Dialogue which deals with the description and interaction of the three categories listed above.

Materials required for administration and scoring are:

1. Tape recording, "Relaxation and Guided Imagery."

2. Drawing materials (8½ x 11" white sheets and reproduction pencils).

3. IMAGE-CA Interview Record and Scoring Sheet.

The manner in which this information is collected is highly contingent upon the patient involved. The patient's

IMAGE-CA
Interview Record and Scoring Sheet

Jeanne Achterberg and G. Frank Lawlis

Biographical/Treatment Data

Age _____   Sex _____   Marital Status _____

Type of Treatment: Date(s):

    Surgery   On _____

    Radiation   from _____ to _____

    Chemotherapy/Immunotherapy   from _____ to _____

    Other   from _____ to _____

Diagnosis: Primary Site _____

                                      Secondary Site(s) _____

Current Disease Status: _____ 1) no evidence of disease

                                          _____ 2) disease stabilized

                                          _____ 3) continued active disease

IMAGE-CA Total Score (sten) _____

Instructions

This booklet is designed for recording and scoring information obtained from patient imagery drawings. After the patient has listened to the guided relaxation exercise, instruct him/her to draw, on a separate 8½ x 11-inch sheet of white paper, (1) the white blood cells, (2) any treatment being received, and (3) the cancer cells, all acting inside the body. When the drawings are completed, begin the interview using pages 3 and 4.

Following the interview, score the imagery/interview content according to the 14 Dimensions appearing on page 2. After scoring each of these scales, fold in page 4 so that **IMAGE CA - Summary Data** (page 5) is directly opposite page 2. Transcribe the 14 scores in column (2) of the table provided on page 5. Next, multiply each of the individual scores by the weights appearing in column (3) and enter the product in column (4). Add these components and enter the sum in the appropriate box marked "Weighted Sum." Then, in the appropriate sten conversion table, find the interval containing the obtained weighted sum and the corresponding sten score.

INSTITUTE FOR PERSONALITY AND ABILITY TESTING

1602-04 Coronado Drive, Champaign, Illinois 61820

FIGURE 3

Circle the number you feel best describes the imagery, based on the information you have available.

CANCER CELLS

	1	2	3	4	5
1. Vividness	very unclear	somewhat unclear	moderately vivid	quite vivid	maximumly vivid
2. Activity	very active	quite active	moderately active	somewhat active	not at all active
3. Strength	very strong	quite strong	moderately strong	moderately weak	quite weak

WHITE BLOOD CELLS (Immune System)

	1	2	3	4	5
4. Vividness	very unclear	somewhat unclear	moderately clear	quite vivid	maximumly vivid
5. Activity	not active	some activity	moderately active	quite active	very active
6. Numerosity (relative to Cancer Cells)	many more Ca than WBC	few more Ca than WBC	about the same WBC & Ca	few more WBC	many more WBC than Ca
7. Size (relative to Cancer Cells)	Ca much larger than WBC	Ca somewhat larger	Ca and WBC about same	WBC little larger	WBC much larger than Ca
8. Strength	quite weak	moderately weak	somewhat strong	quite strong	very strong

TREATMENT (Circle "3" if patient is not receiving treatment)

	1	2	3	4	5
9. Vividness	very unclear, confused	somewhat unclear	moderately clear	quite vivid	very vivid, clear
10. Effectiveness	not at all effective	moderately ineffective	moderately effective	quite effective	highly effective

GENERAL

	1	2	3	4	5
11. How Symbolistic is visualization vs. How Concrete	very factual, concrete	moderately factual, concrete	mixed symbolistic/ factual	moderately symbolistic	highly symbolistic
12. Overall Strength of Imagery vs. Weakness	very weak	quite weak	moderate	quite strong	very sound, strong
13. Estimated regularity	not imaging	infrequent	moderately regular	high level of consistency	extremely frequent
14. In your opinion, how is this type of imagery related to short-term disease management	continued active disease	some stabilization	considerable stabilization	eventual remission	rapid remission

FIGURE 3 (Continued)

Cancer
   1. Describe how your cancer cells look in your mind's eye.

   2. Do you see the cancer cells moving around? If so, how? When?

   3. How strong (tough) do you think your cells are? (Score on strength described or imputed to symbol chosen).

White Blood Cells [WBC]
   4. Describe your WBC. (Score on vividness, clarity, continuity of description).

   5. Do you see your WBC moving? If so, how? Where? (Score on activity or potential activity of symbol).

   6. Do you see more cancer or more WBC? (Scoring on obvious response).

FIGURE 3 (Continued)

7. How big are your cancer cells? Your white blood cells?* (Score on relative difference with "5" indicating WBC significantly larger).

8. *How* do the WBC fight disease in your body? How well do you see the WBC as doing their job? (Score on strength or effectiveness).

Treatment
9. How does your treatment work to rid your body of disease? (Score on clarity and vividness).

10. How *well* does your treatment work to kill off disease? (Score on effectiveness described).

Miscellaneous Response
11. (Score on symbolism vs. concretion).

12. (Score on weak vs. strong).

13. How many times a day do you think about (or image) your cancer? (Record response).

14. (Score imagery on basis of how you would predict it related to disease from a clinical standpoint, i.e., "5" would indicate it predicted complete recovery, a "1" would predict a poor prognosis or death).

---

*Patient may be confused on difference between cancer *cell* and *tumor*. If so, some explanation or rewording may be required.

FIGURE 3 (Continued)

IMAGE-CA - Summary Data *

(1)	(2)	(3)	(4)
Dimension	Score x Weight	=	Weighted Score
1	_____ x 1		_____
2	_____ x 1		_____
3	_____ x 3		_____
4	_____ x 3		_____
5	_____ x 4		_____
6	_____ x 1		_____
7	_____ x 3		_____
8	_____ x 4		_____
9	_____ x 2		_____
10	_____ x 3		_____
11	_____ x 1		_____
12	_____ x 6		_____
13	_____ x 1		_____
14	_____ x 16		_____

➤ ☐ Weighted Sum Without Dimension 14 (see Columns 5a and 6a below)

➤ ☐ Weighted Sum With Dimension 14 (see Columns 5b and 6b below)

Sten Conversion Table
For Use With Only 13 Dimensions
(omitting clinical judgment, Dimension 14)

(5a) Weighted Sum	(6a) Sten	
165 or greater	10	Excellent imagery
153-162	9	
144-152	8	Good imagery
134-143	7	
125-133	6	Average imagery
115-124	5	
106-114	4	Less than average
96-105	3	imagery
87- 95	2	Poor imagery
less than 86	1	

Sten Conversion Table
For Use With All 14 Dimensions

(5b) Weighted Sum	(6b) Sten	
247 or greater	10	Excellent imagery
229-246	9	
213-228	8	Good imagery
195-212	7	
178-194	6	Average imagery
161-177	5	
144-160	4	Less than average
127-143	3	imagery
110-126	2	Poor imagery
less than 109	1	

* **Note:** For individuals with relatively little experience using the IMAGE-CA drawing technique (less than 50 administrations), omission of Dimension 14 is advised. Therefore, the sten conversion table on the left of this page should be used. For a more detailed explanation of scoring procedures, see pp. 85-89, *Imagery of Cancer: An evaluation tool for the process of disease*, Achterberg & Lawlis, 1978.

FIGURE 3 (Continued)

physical condition is of primary consideration. The manner of administration will differ greatly depending upon whether a patient is ambulatory or bedridden, highly medicated or alert, inpatient or outpatient, and so forth. We encountered patients at every conceivable stage of disease, socioeconomic level, and motivational state. The variables involved in a patient's willingness and ability to perform must be dealt with on an individual basis. The usual format for administration will be given below and includes (1) listening to a relaxation and guided imagery tape, (2) drawing the visualizations, and (3) a structured interview.

Relaxation and Guided Imagery Instructions

All patients on whom IMAGE-CA was developed had some exposure to an audio tape recording which began with relaxation exercises, and was followed by information on imaging the cancer, the immune system, and any treatment that was being administered. One group of patients (Normative Group I) had listened to a tape produced by Carl Simonton (Special recording, Cognetics, Inc.) three times daily for a minimum of two weeks prior to their first session. The Medical School/county hospital patients (Normative Group II) were exposed to another audio tape only once immediately prior to administration of the IMAGE-CA. A transcript of this tape, developed primarily for this evaluation instrument follows:

Transcription of the Cancer Evaluation Tape

This is a tape that will help you relax your body and understand your disease a little better. First of all, I would like for you to be sitting in a way that you can be very relaxed and very comfortable. You may wish to lie down. I will give you a few seconds to situate yourself in your chair, on your bed, so that your arms and legs can be relaxed and comfortable, and so that your back can be supported. Now, I would like for you to pick a spot on the wall, comfortably look at it, and as I count downwards from 10, I want you to continue to stare at the spot, until your eyes become very heavy. 10, 9, 8, 7, 6, 5, 4, 3, 2, 1. Now, gently close your eyes, and ignore all the sounds outside of the room. Just concentrate on my voice. Take some very deep breaths, breathing slowly and deeply, letting the air come in and go out. Each time you breathe out, let some of the tension leave your body. Breathe in; breathe out; say to yourself, relax. Let that relaxed feeling spread all over your body. Now, think for a moment about your feet. Let all of the tension flow out of your feet. Let the muscles become very loose and very smooth; very warm. Imagine the blood warming your feet, making them tingly. Think for a moment about your legs, your lower legs, your calves. Let all the tension dissolve out of them, melting away, making them soft and smooth. Your upper legs, your thighs, let them become very warm. Now, at the count of 3 I would like you to be twice as relaxed as you are now. 1, 2, 3. In your mind's eye, concentrate for a moment on your hips, letting them come very loose; muscles in your abdomen— where you may be storing a lot of tension—let that go. Let the blood flow through like the wind through the wheat, carrying good oxygen to all of your body. Continue to breathe regularly and deeply. Think for a second about the many muscles in your back. Mentally tell them to relax, to let go of all tension and stress and anxiety that they may be showing. Imagine the tension knots in your back and in your shoulders dissolving, melting, going away. The muscles in your neck, relax— become very soft—just let them go. All up and down the back of your head and the top of your head, let the tension free, flowing out. Allow the tiny muscles around your eyes to relax, around your jaw. Now, if you are still feeling pain or tension in some part of your body, I'm going to pause for a moment and let you concentrate on that area.

Pause.

35

Now, while your body is quiet and you are in touch with it, I would like to remind you that the body is like a marvelous machine. It has built-in devices for protecting itself. It has white blood cells that attack and kill the danger cells that enter into it. These danger cells might be cancer cells or some other abnormal cells. Normally, the white blood cells help to protect your body against cancer and other diseases. Remind yourself that within your body, right now, are cells that are very, very powerful. I want you to imagine these, see them becoming active, guarding you, protecting you. See them doing it very, very well. See your white blood cells, any way that makes sense to you, attacking all abnormal cells; attacking the tumor. See them doing their job, like experts, destroying the cancer cells, keeping your body healthy and disease-free. And, now, if you are still receiving some kind of treatment, x-ray or chemotherapy, I want you to see that treatment working effectively inside of your body. I want you to see it operating together with your white blood cells to allow you to return to health; to maintain your health. Remember that when your body is relaxed, like it should be now, your defenses against disease are better, and you are better able to participate with your medical treatment. I would like for you to see yourself being the kind of person that you want to be, doing the things that have meaning for you, achieving and maintaining health. And, I would like for you to congratulate yourself for having spent a few minutes allowing your body to relax and allowing it to function in the best way possible. Now, in a moment I'm going to ask you to draw, in any way that you wish, your thoughts about what you have been imagining and pretending, to see on a journey inside of your body; about your white blood cells, about your treatment, and about your cancer. Now, first, I want you to remember to just relax and to feel good about yourself. I'm going to count to 3, and at the count of 3, I want you to gently open your eyes and begin to listen for the next instructions. 1, 2, 3.

It is fairly obvious that the presentation of the tape has therapeutic implications, even if the patients do not use it on a regular basis. First, some methods of relaxation are offered which presumably produce residual physical benefit, particularly if the patient chooses to adopt them in some fashion at a later time. They may well do so since the benefits of relaxation as an aid to health are spelled out. Second, new information is given to the patient which may be helpful in evoking an attitude change, such as the notion of a surveillance system, a built-in system of defense, and the natural process of healing. Finally, suggestions are provided for cooperation with medical treatment, much of which is quite aversive to the patients and is met with dread and tension which no doubt accentuates side effects.

The tape that is included with the IMAGE-CA has been tested on patients with reading levels as low as second grade, as well as on patients with professional educational attainments. The tape, and indeed the procedure itself, appears to be valid on adult patients with reading levels as low as 4th grade (but not lower). If some mental retardation or brain damage is suspected, we recommend the Ohio Literacy Test. Reported educational levels were not found to correlate with reading levels at the lower end of the spectrum, and hence are not too useful here. Obviously, patients with certain primary or metastatic brain tumors will have difficulty in processing the information required and the validity is questionable. Many such patients appeared to comprehend the taped instructions and benefit from the relaxation exercises nevertheless.

The tape designed for the test is significantly different from the tapes produced by Simonton on virtually every feature except for the overall format of relaxation instructions, together with a discussion for the imaging of the disease, treatment, and immune system. The Simonton tape is designed for regular therapeutic use and patient education and is approximately 18 minutes in length. The relaxation portion on the most recent version lasts 4 minutes, whereas the IMAGE-CA tape relaxation portion lasts 12 minutes and contains more specific suggestions on breathing and on imaging the muscles relaxing.

The Simonton version offers guided imagery suggestions for visualizing the disease, treatment, and immune system components. For example, the suggestion is made to see the cancer as "raw hamburger or liver," "a weak, confused cell," "a blackened area," and the radiation as "millions of bullets of energy," and an explanation is provided for the mode of action of chemotherapy. The IMAGE-CA evaluation tape, on the other hand, attempts to skirt the issue of image programming by not providing specific suggestions.

The Drawings

Patients are requested to draw on 8½ x 11-inch white paper a picture which contains three things: (1) their tumors (or disease, or cancer) as they picture it in their mind's eye; (2) their body's defense against the tumor, or the white blood cells; and (3) their treatment, if any is being received. Frequently, the patients will protest that they cannot draw. It is a good idea to assure these patients that detail, not artistic ability, is what is sought.

A rule of thumb concerning length of time for the drawing is to remember that nothing is to be gained by rushing a patient through the exercise—incomplete drawings waste everyone's time. Again, the patient's situation must be taken into account. Patients who were being given psychotherapy in a week-long residential type setting were allowed to take home several sheets of paper and asked to bring the pictures in the following day. On the other hand, outpatients attending a cancer clinic were requested to complete them during the testing session.

Patients are asked to use reproduction pens or pencils to do the drawings. We are frequently asked why we do not provide colors, since some interesting effects would doubtlessly transpire. We agree. Patients in residence frequently found colors and used them despite the fact that many were living out of suitcases in a motel! There is, in fact, evidence from Bruno Klopfer's work (1957) on the Rorschach that cancer patients have peculiarities in using colors, interestingly enough, and we heartily endorse the extended development of the IMAGE-CA to include this variable. However, it was not consonant with our initial goal of simplifying the complexities of the imagery studies.

The Dialogue

After having completed the drawing, the patient is asked to discuss the three factors that were drawn. Both patient and evaluator should have access to the drawing at this point.

For the bulk of patients, a structured interview format is suggested in order to assure that all the appropriate items will be covered. To this end, a series of questions was developed, and appears on pages 3 and 4 of the IMAGE-CA Interview Record and Scoring Sheet (see Fig. 3). The questions merely form the skeletal basis for the interview procedure. As with any projective instrument, the skill of the administrator is a major determinant of the amount of clinical information that is obtained. (We will discuss the actual scoring procedures and the remainder of the scoring booklet in sections dealing with evaluating the imagery, p. 50.)

Methods for obtaining dialogue may vary for experienced interviewers. The patients who had been involved in a regular relaxation/imagery procedure for several weeks were given 7 minutes to recite the content of their imagery and notes of the dialogue were made by an evaluator. At the termination of the recitation, specific questions were asked in order to gain information on any item on the 14-item scoring sheet that may have been omitted. This procedure was used because the patients were in a group therapy mileu, and the time limit was necessary to allow all patients to have an opportunity for discussion and critique. For patients who are involved in a regular imagery procedure there is virtue in replicating this set of circumstances for data collection, because it allows the patient freedom to go through a recapitulation of the procedure, and valuable information can be offered, based on the more subtle cues of voice inflection and the emotional investment in images.

The patient's responses should be carefully recorded on the Interview Record so that appropriate evaluation may be made after the session. It is quite valuable to tape record the interview session and to transcribe or preserve the tapes so that they form a part of the patient's permanent record, particularly when naive or novice interviewers are used to gather the data.

We have included two examples of skilled interviewing conducted by Donna Kelly-Powell and Harriett Gibbs. The first interview was confined to the questioning procedure and is directed and highly structured. The second was more expansive, primarily because of the investigators' desires to extend the interview to peripheral areas that revealed a great deal about the management of the patient's disease.

Sample Dialogue I: A directed, highly structured approach

Interviewer: Can you describe to me what those cancer cells look like?
Patient: I would imagine they were a massive, moldy thing.
I: Not just the tumor, but the individual cancer cells?
P: Imagine a very irregular shape for the cancer cells.
I: What about size of the irregular shape?
P: Small, about the size of a pinhead.
I: Do they have colors?
P: Dark colors.
I: Do you see them moving around at all?
P: Milling or pulsating is a better word.
I: Where are they moving to?
P: They are just marking time.
I: What are they marking time for?
P: I don't know.
I: How strong do they appear to be?
P: Not very.
I: Kind of weak?
P: That would be a good word.

I: Now tell me about your white blood cells, can you see your white blood cells, what do they look like?

P: They are sort of bean-shaped and little on each end and kind of fat in the middle.

I: Why do you think they are shaped that way?

P: Because that's what I was taught in school.

I: Can you see any color to them at all?

P: No.

I: Do you see those moving around?

P: Yes. They travel around all the time.

I: How do they travel?

P: In the bloodstream, to the source of any infection or disease, all the time.

I: Picture again your cancer cells and your white blood cells, both of them, which of them is bigger?

P: The white blood cells are bigger than the cancer cell, not the mass, but the cell.

I: Which do you see more of, the cancer cells or white blood cells?

P: The white blood cells.

I: About how many more do you see?

P: Twice as many.

I: How well do you see those white blood cells as doing their job?

P: Quite well.

I: Are they fighting with the cancer?

P: Engulfing it would be a better word.

I: Do you see them as winning over or losing? How are they doing?

P: Winning.

I: Let's move onto a different picture about the treatment that you receive. What type of treatment did you get?

P: Radiation.

I: Can you picture that? How do you feel that the radiation has worked inside your body to help rid your body of the disease you have?

41

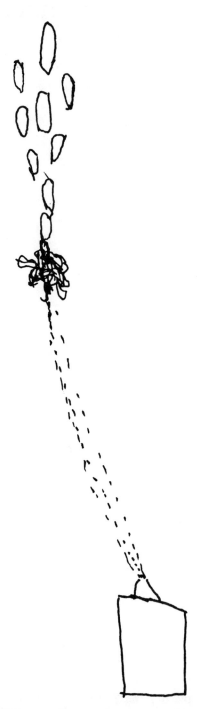

FIGURE 4. WHITE BLOOD CELLS AND RADIATION ATTACKING
RESIDUAL TUMOR CELLS FROM BREAST MASS (DIALOGUE I)

P: A destruction type of remedy, destroying the cells.

I: How were they destroying it?

P: By radiation.

I: How would you say the radiation was destroying the cancer cells?

P: Doing away with; wiping out; destruction.

I: Do you see the cancer cells as disappearing? How well do you feel that radiation treatment is working to kill the disease?

P: Well, I think it completely got rid of the disease.

I: How many times a day do you think about your cancer and having had cancer?

P: Days go by and I never ever think about it. Very rarely.

I: Would you say maybe once a week?

P: If that often.

I: It may be every two weeks before you even think about it at all?

P: Yes.

I: Open your eyes and look at this picture and describe it to me.

P: The blood cells going after the cancer and the radiation coming down.

I: This is the cancer and this is the white blood cells? (See Figure 4.)

P: Yes.

Sample Dialogue II: An expansive approach

Interviewer: What did your cancer cell look like in your mind's eye when you were relaxed?

Patient: I would say it was sort of a light brown cell with a structure of little nodes inside and the white corpuscle. . . .

I: Wait, let's not leave the cancer cell yet, you said it was brown?

43

P: Light brown with a blister-like appearance.

I: Does it look big or small?

P: It's relatively small.

I: Is it a tough thing?

P: No, it's a membrane and it's not tough at all, in fact, if it wasn't brown you could see through it, be transparent.

I: The stuff inside, what's it made of?

P: It's sort of like the pericardium of the heart, it's like enveloped with a fluid.

I: Can we call that a jelly-like substance?

P: Yes.

I: Does it move around?

P: Oh yes.

I: Can you describe that for me? What does this cell do?

P: Just like a bed of ants, constantly never stopping, but I think a lot of them are consumed by these white corpuscles.

I: When does it move? Where is it going?

P: Just over the body.

I: All over the body?

P: Yes, every place in the muscles, in the tissues. But the good thing about it I guess, is where they can go the white corpuscles can go too.

I: So they don't go somewhere that the treatment or the white cells can't get to it?

P: That's right.

I: When does it move, when is it most active?

P: I'd say it is when you're least active.

I: How does it move, does it have arms?

P: No, there's an involvement there that it moves with, wherever it wants to, just like your blood, it can be a part of your bloodstream. It can get into certain areas, the kidneys, bladder, into the different parts of the body.

I: You know how you beautifully described your cancer cell for me? Let's do the same for the white blood cell now.

P: It's around the same as a cancer cell—in fact the way I depicted a cancer cell was a white corpuscle and something happened to it, I don't know what, it wasn't raised up right, it turned bad and multiplied and they multiply fast. The white corpuscle has the ability to work like a muscle, they can open up and devour the cancer cells, they feed off them then as they kill the cancer cells out in certain sections those white corpuscles are no use to the body anymore and the body has to continue to make new white blood cells. That is why it is of the utmost importance that a cancer patient be instructed on a diet so the body can continue to make these white cells.

I: Describe the white cell for me like you did the cancer cell. What kind of appearance does it have? Does it have a color?

P: It's white in looks and of a jelly-like substance, but it can open up, in other words if there is something that's not right in the body it can defend it.

I: Do you see it as having special arms or any special apparatus to do that?

P: No, just muscle.

I: Just muscle, how does it do it? Does it surround the cell?

P: Yes.

I: Tell me, are there more white blood cells than cancer cells?

P: Well, no there's not. If there were I have a feeling there'd be less cancer. It's according to the patient.

I: What do you think you have?

P: Well, I don't think I have cancer.

I: What does that mean?

P: I think I have been cured.

I: Does that mean you think you have a whole lot of white blood cells?

P: I don't think I have really enough, don't misunderstand me, there's been an illness here and in any illness there's going to be a breakdown of the body as the cancer patient builds these white corpuscles up it seems like there's not enough to envelop all the cancer cells because the cancer cells do multiply fast.

I: Who do you see as winning?

P: I believe I'm going to win.

45

I: So you think even though the white blood cells may be out-numbered they can still take care of the cancer cells?

P: Well, we have to go back to religion and belief. I prayed and it's a matter of soul searching and having the belief that God can do this and I do believe that he has healed me. Now I have aches and pains, but I believe it's due to arthritis, it might fool me, but I'm saying I believe this. I believe that the key is in going about your daily living and helping other people.

I: Getting your mind off yourself and on someone else.

P: That's it, helping other people that's 99% of cancer treatment, I do believe.

I: Let's go back for a bit to a couple of other things about the white blood cell. Are they big in your mind's eye?

P: Yes.

I: Are they bigger than the cancer cell?

P: Yes, about twice as big.

I: Do these white blood cells move around?

P: Yes they do, to an extent but not like cancer cells. In my thought a white corpuscle will devour the cancer cell and it's like they can take so much of eating cancer cells and then they're like elephants, they go over here to a certain spot and collect together because their work is done. They can become like a big sore, sometimes they just burst.

I: In other words once they have done all they can do to fight these cancer cells they collect together and the body gets rid of them?

P: In time, and if the body doesn't get rid of them they can get in the tissues, rot, and that in turn causes a body to sour, the person emits in their breath, in the body, sort of a dead smell. They will collect in the body like a big boil and burst and have to come out, it's in the form of pus, all the cancer cells and corpuscles.

I: When the white cells leave they take the cancer cells with them?

P: Yes, those cancer cells are devoured and I think that's what in my mind would create all the pus and stuff.

46

I: When are these white corpuscles the most active?

P: They're active all the time, but the body just doesn't have enough of them. We've got to be on a strict diet in order for the body to make the cells. Then after they're made, you see, cancer isn't the only thing the white corpuscle has to contend with, they have other diseases they have to handle. It's a pretty good job they have to do.

I: Do you see them as doing a good job?

P: Yes, but it's so hard to get a cancer patient to eat right after treatment. I think you've got to get someone who's been there. I believe if people would be more attentive, encouraging them, showing they're interested in them, that they care, well that's the biggest part of the ball game.

I: You should be able to handle cancer with the proper diet and right thinking?

P: I believe you can delay it even if it is inevitable that cancer is going to take you. I believe your attitude and the right way of thinking can postpone that. I have faith and believe it.

I: Can you describe how you see your treatment working? (Looking at drawing; see Figure 5.) First of all what are the black dots?

P: That was the cancer cell. They were burned to a degree that there's no way that the ones left after surgery are alive. This is the scorched burned area that the radiation caused. This up here is the dead cells.

I: Why are they dead?

P: Because of the treatment.

I: Do you have any picture of what the treatment looks like when it hits the tumor?

P: It's sort of a blast.

I: Is there a color to it? Can you describe it?

P: Yes, there is a color to it, it's so penetrating. I believe it would be so intense; well, a ultraviolet light would be purple, I just believe it's so penetrating that it doesn't have color.

I: So it's just an intense beam or blast of some sort.

P: Yes.

I: And it hits these cells that were over there and what does it do to them?

P: Well, it wastes them to where they don't have the mobility to attack the brain. I believe it's all wasted away during this time. There's also the chance that some of these brown ones can get a free ride in the bloodstream to other parts of the body.

I: These brown ones have been burned?

P: Yes.

I: Have they lost their power?

P: Yes, they've lost their power.

I: How did the treatment kill them?

P: The ray was so intense, you know nothing can live under that, I couldn't if I was to have to.

I: So you saw the treatment as being very powerful?

P: Yes.

I: And effective?

P: Yes, I would say it's effective. I wouldn't want any more of it. I've had quite enough. When a cancer patient goes through this phase of treatment a lot of them like me can't comprehend it's me, me having cancer, having a tumor, just when I thought I had the world by the tail. I said well, old devil like to got me, so I just changed my way of thinking and got my attitude changed, my appearance changed overnight and my whole life changed all the way around and I'm all the better for it.

(Back to drawing for summing up.)

I: This is the cancer cell by itself. This bean-shaped body is the white blood cell.

P: Yes, these are the cancer cells. These (WBC) are just as round as these in appearance but they can open up their muscle and eat the cancer.

I: They're in their open state here encircling this body?

P: Yes.

I: These little brown specks are what's left over after it's eaten.

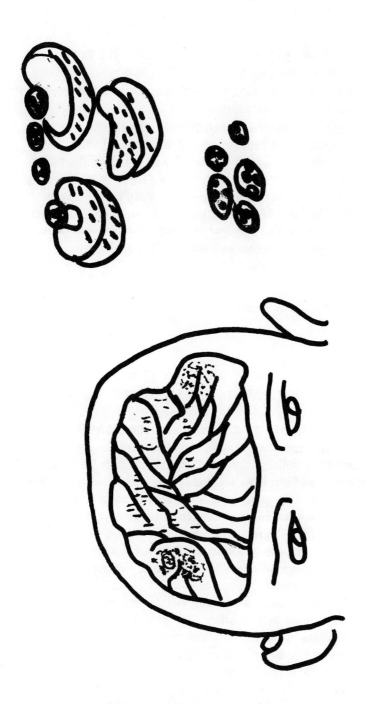

FIGURE 5. WHITE BLOOD CELLS AND METASTATIC BRAIN
CANCER (DIALOGUE II)

P: That's a Walt Disney opinion of it (laughs). It's hard to put it down in words.

I: When you were thinking in your imagination, how clearly did you see this in your mind?

P: I thought of a show I'd seen (movie—Fantastic Voyage). They miniaturized these men and inject them into a vein. That instantly came to my mind—I was going up the blood-stream looking into the area of the intestine and seeing these white corpuscles and how they didn't have any path in mind, but they were moving and they bounced, and each time they could take a cancer cell and devour it and bounce down here and open this side up and do it again.

I: Sounds like it goes pretty fast.

P: Oh, yes.

I: You saw that very clearly?

P: I did.

EVALUATING THE IMAGERY

Scores for the 14 dimensions of the IMAGE-CA are derived from the two types of information previously described: (1) the drawings, and (2) the records of dialogue from structured interview sessions. It is valuable to observe at the onset that frequently there may be no precise statement or figure that corresponds to a particular dimension. However, the high degree of interrater agreement obtained in the norming studies on all factors of the protocol indicates that reliable ratings can be given based on the overall context of the imagery described.

The dimensions were derived from careful study of the imagery described in over 200 patient sessions. They represent points of discussion which patients themselves most frequently used to describe their imagined physical condition. Scoring the IMAGE-CA involves a degree of subjective impression, some familiarity with the disease, and sensitivity to the personality of the cancer patient. Its utility as a predictive device should, therefore, increase as the clinician gains expertise in these areas. Clinically, however, it has immediate value in aiding the researcher or the therapist in focusing on facets of the patient's attitude toward disease that have been shown to correlate either positively or negatively with the course of the malignancy. Ultimately, it offers guidelines for the clinician in aiding the patient to adopt more positive attitudes toward recovery.

The individual dimensions on the IMAGE-CA are discussed in the sections that follow. The rationale for the inclusion of each scale and examples of scoring strategies are also included. The statistical characteristics of the scales will be treated in finer detail in a later section.

The 14 scoring dimensions appear on page 2 of the IMAGE-CA Interview Record and Scoring Sheet (Please refer to Figure 3, p. 30). Judgments based on both drawings and dialogue/interviews are combined to derive the scores. Each factor is rated on a scale of five points, with (1) generally considered weak or ineffective and (5) considered as strong or most desirable. The total IMAGE-CA score is simply the sum of the points obtained on each of the 14 dimensions.

The system for evaluating the imagery or disease has three natural divisions: (1) The Disease (Cancer); (2) The Body's Defenses or Immunity (White Blood Cells); and (3) Treatment (in the case of cancer would usually be radiation, chemotherapy, immunotherapy, surgery, or a combination of these). A fourth division in the analysis of imagery relates to the more subtle cues that are imparted by the patient to the therapist or researcher, and which allow the inclusion of clinical judgment based on less definable, but nevertheless important factors. Each of the items identified below should be considered after carefully reviewing the patient's statement, and with a clear notion of the configuration of the patient's drawings. When the drawings are vague or imprecise, the dialogue may provide the only source of information on which judgments may be formed. On the other hand, with insufficient questioning (or in cases where patients may be either low verbal or aphasic), suppositions are based exclusively on the drawing. However, in most cases we found that when questioning was accomplished according to the format described in the previous section, and when patients

51

were given sufficient time and encouragement to complete the drawings, there was good congruence between them, and virtually all of the information required to complete the scoring sheet could be obtained in one way or another.

After each of the individual disease dimensions has been assigned a scale score of 1—5, a total score is obtained as follows. First, transpose each of the 14 scores to the Summary Data table provided on page 5 of the Interview Record and Scoring Sheet (Figure 3). Next, multiply each of these scores by the weights contained in column (3) of this table to yield weighted scores (in column (4)). By summing these components, one derives a "weighted sum." Finally, a total sten score is derived by locating the weighted sum in the sten conversion tables located on the bottom of page 5 of the scoring booklet. The total sten score can then be entered in the boxes provided on the front page of the scoring booklet for easy reference and comparisons with scores obtained in subsequent administrations. The reader will notice that a "weighted sum" may be derived using either 13 or 14 dimensions. Individuals with relatively little experience using the IMAGE-CA (less than 50 administrations) are advised to omit Dimension 14, the overall clinical evaluation.

In the following section only relevant and composite portions of the drawings are presented, together with an abbreviated dialogue. In all cases the anonymity of the patient has been respected. Here, and in all case history discussions, disease status and other criteria are based on follow-up information obtained approximately 6 months after initial data collection.

DISEASE DIMENSIONS

Dimension 1: Vividness of cancer cells

For this first scale, vividness or clarity of the description is used as the criterion for judgment. Here, the relevant question the researcher should ask is whether from the patient's description a clear image is conveyed of the way the patient sees his tumor. This item was relatively less important than others as a predictor of short-term disease state, but it was retained because of the information it offers on the general ability of the patient to image. In this regard it contributes to the overall validity of the instrument scoring system and serves as a logical initial focus to begin the analysis.

It was frequently observed that patients who were very sick or who suffered recurrent disease in the short-run were able to vividly describe their cancer cells, but were unable to formulate a clear impression of the treatment or immune response. Not surprisingly, a large portion of the drawings of many of the indigent patients was devoted to the cancer cell. Detail was more complete and dialogue was more readily obtained than similar events regarding the white blood cell. It stands to reason that since disease condition is more prominent and more familiar to patients, it would be more vividly described than an immune mechanism which they may know little about and may indeed have little trust in after a diagnosis of malignancy. To reiterate, the vividness of imagery of the cancer cell was not strongly related to disease response and primarily serves to bring the task into focus.

An example of a patient whose imagery was scored "5," or extremely vivid on the disease factor, is presented in Figure 6. Both in terms of the appearance of the cell and the dynamics of interaction, the description comes across extremely clear. This case presents an interesting situation, since based on every indication available including experience as a visual imager, the patient was able to form quite vivid images, yet the description is most definitely not one congruent with a positive attitude toward a return to health.

A low score on this factor is rare, but may come about in any of several ways. Low verbal adult patients (usually those with a reading level of 4th grade or lower) or patients who were unable to comprehend the test because of brain involvement would present a vague description. Generally in these cases the validity of the IMAGE-CA is questionable. A low score on this variable might also occur when a patient erroneously believes that the cancer is no longer there, or refuses to acknowledge the existence of disease. An example

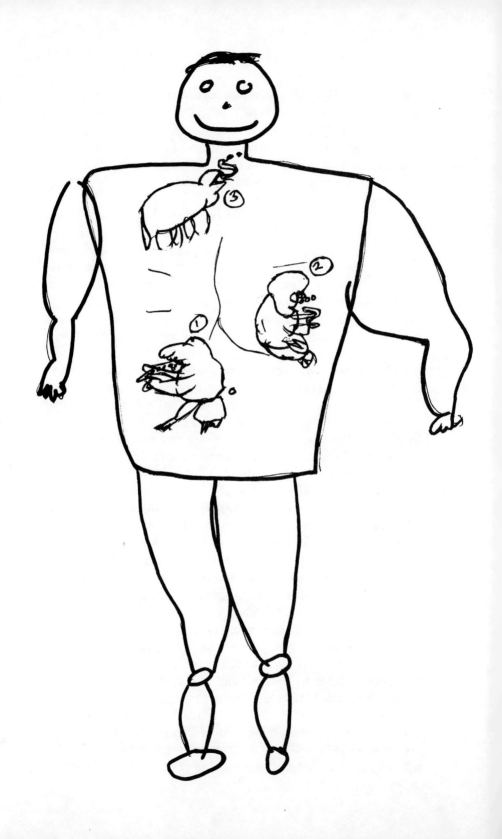

FIGURE 6. IMAGERY SCORED HIGH ON VIVIDNESS OF DISEASE (DIMENSION 1)

*The patient relaxes himself three times daily, for
5-15 minutes each time. His relaxation consists of taking
deep breaths, counting backwards, and going over muscle
groups. His liver is described as a small snake, curled
around itself two or three times. Chemotherapy goes to
liver, lung, and neck and is seen as a white spray
hitting the snake. The immune system is a polar bear,
and the bear tears the snake apart. Sometimes, however,
the snake is automatically transformed into a duck or
some other friendly animal. Sometimes it becomes an
airplane. The patient describes feeling actual streams of cold
or hot activity in his body. In describing the immune
system, he says these bears put their paw or tongue
in his clavicle, and work their way through the body
to the lung, liver, and hip. Occasionally, the snake is in
water and this impairs the efficiency of the bears. He
ends his imagery seeing himself healthy and walking on the
beach. He says he feels he has actually done something
with his imagery, but not activated the immune system.
He also said that when he loses emotional control, he feels
he loses physical control in regard to cellular growth.*

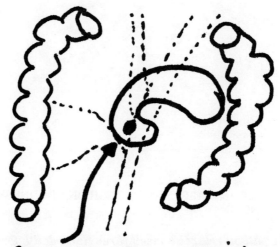

Dehydrated residue
of carcinoma on
the head of the
Pancreas

FIGURE 7. IMAGERY SCORED LOW ON VIVIDNESS OF DISEASE (DIMENSION 1). PATIENT DENIES EXISTENCE OF CANCER, DESPITE MEDICAL EVIDENCE TO CONTRARY

The patient regards chemotherapy as a continuous cleansing agent. He does not picture himself as having any cancer currently. Earlier, he saw his tumor as a hard, solid mass with no protrusions. The radiation affected it rapidly, serving as an energy source. He said the cancer is now dry and crusted, but is no longer living. The pancreas, he believed, was rebuilding. When questioned more about his chemotherapy, he said he had no real visualization for it, but that it may simply stir up the white blood cells. He does not envision any rebuilding process occurring nor any other action between the white blood cells and cancer cells. He says in his imagination he cleanses himself with a sprayer, focusing on any pain. The spray is green soap. He has a vacuum cleaner that works on his stomach, cleaning out the soap and any foreign matter. He reiterated that he has no cancer cells now and that he is angry because he feels he should not be having a reaction and pain that he now has.

of this kind of denial is presented in Figure 7. Medical records for this individual indicated active disease, and the patient had been informed accordingly by the physician. Frequently, in using this technique with a patient, there may indeed be no reason to suspect the presence of active cancer (this was true particularly in a group of breast cancer patients included in Normative Group II—many of whom had recent mastectomies). In these cases the patients are asked to recall how the disease appeared prior to surgery. Interestingly, the scores obtained in this manner on the cancer portion were as well distributed as those from patients who were currently being treated for disease.

Dimension 2: Activity of the cancer cells

The second factor relating to the imagery of the cancer cell itself is that of activity. It was selected because of the belief that movement or activity would imply growth or metastasis in the system, and would tap the patient's attitude toward spread of the malignancy. During the sessions there was a high frequency of remarks such as "I can feel the cells crawling down my legs and arms," or "Sometimes when I'm sitting quietly, I can actually feel movement in the tumor area." Since cancer patients are prone to "second-guess" any unusual physical sensation as tumor spread, the factor may be an indirect measure of the anxiety level a patient has regarding recurrent disease. The scale is designed so that the more active or the more *potential* activity the patient attributes to the tumor, the lower the rating. Thus a quiescent description is given a "5" and an exceedingly active depiction receives a "1." Not only is the patient's description of the tumor's activity taken into account (i.e., "it moves sluggish, like a snail," or "fast as lightning"), but also the type of activity that can be imputed to the symbol chosen. Frequently, patients will describe the cancer as animals, which are certainly capable of movement of varying degrees, as compared with descriptions of tumors as blobs or bubbles which have more inert properties.

For example, the drawing in Figure 8 uses the symbology of submarines to represent the cancer cells. This aspect received a low rating, since the ships imply the ability to move. More so, perhaps, they imply a mysteriousness to the movement; an unpredictability; a constant wariness and wondering about the next point of emergency. The crab, a frequently chosen symbol in all groups studied, was also given generally low ratings because of the implications of movement and the unpredictability of the response. On the other hand, the use of an animal such as a slug would imply slow or reduced activity, particularly when used in contrast with the active, powerful wolves or dogs representing the white blood cells.

Dimension 3: Strength of cancer cells

The strength of the disease described during the questioning procedure or the potential strength that can be attributed to the image chosen by the patient is used to determine the rating on this scale. This particular factor has been shown to be the most important of the three cancer cell ratings in predicting subsequent disease. The more powerful or immutable the object, the "harder" or tougher the symbol chosen, the less the patient may feel that his cancer is capable of being diminished. Also, it stands to reason that a patient who views the tumor as nondestructible may be less willing to fight to overcome the disease. This scale, which basically represents the patient's attitude toward conquerability of the disease, requires some sensitivity in judgment, since the strength of the image is very much determined by the context of the entire representation.

High scores on this factor are given to potentially fragile or readily destructible images; low scores to images which are strong and hence undesirable from a disease standpoint. Again, the image of the submarine described in Case 2 would be given a low score (1) for several reasons: (1) It is made of metal and constructed to be virtually indestructible; (2) it has power and strength as a vehicle of war; and (3) of prime importance, its comparative strength is excessive. (In this case the WBC were described as attacking by shooting pellets, which would not normally affect the structure.) In contrast, a high or positive score would be given to cancer

59

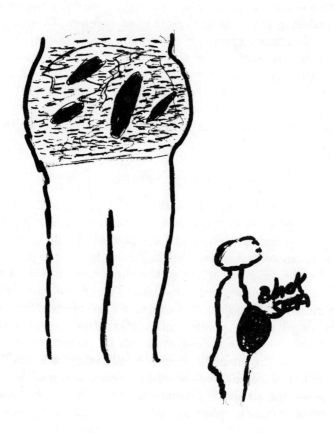

FIGURE 8. LOW RATING ON ACTIVITY OF CANCER CELLS
(DIMENSION 2)

The patient says that he spends a lot of time imaging the fluid in his stomach. He feels that he should be getting to the source or cause of the fluid rather than just working on it, per se. He images his chemotherapy going to his abdomen. He sees his cancer as large masses, all different sizes. The biggest is about the size of a fist, and all of them look like black submarines. The white blood cells attack them and sometimes they score while sometimes they miss and are annihilated. They look like little pellets going into the cancer. The cancer is funneled through a canal. When asked what kills the cancer, the patient said his white blood cells explode and kill thousands of the cancer cells, but there are far too many. Chemotherapy was described as a fluid, greenish in color, which mixes with the fluid in his abdomen. He says he has no clearer picture of this, and has had no side effects from his treatment.

symbols which are soft or particularly destructible in the context used.

In evaluating the imagery of patients who chose more anatomically valid representations, the same criteria for strength hold. Key phrases such as "they no longer have nuclei" indicate their source of nourishment or integration is removed. Descriptions such as "delicate," or as "collapsing," when exposed to treatment would also indicate low imaged strength.

THE BODY'S DEFENSES

Dimension 4: Vividness of white blood cells

As with Dimension 1 (Vividness of cancer cells), this rating is based on how definite a picture the evaluator can obtain of the patient's imagery of the white blood cells. The ratings on this factor (as with all items involving the white blood cells except Dimension 6) are generally more important in determining short-term outcome of disease than the imagery involving the cancer cell, per se. It is our feeling that the white blood cells usually are symbols on which the patients project much of their own belief system regarding the ability to overcome the disease. A few patients will neglect any description of the white blood cells, regardless of the instructions given to them. Several of our subjects simply fell silent and refused to respond to our requests to discuss this phenomena. Often they became anxious and asked to move on to another topic. It is most important to note these cases. If, indeed, the imagery associated with the white blood cells represents the attitude the patients hold regarding their control over the disease, and if they fail to describe this adequately, it may well mean they feel defenseless or victimized by the disease, with little hope of recovery. Such a patient is described in detail in the section on "The Patients" (p. 97. See also, Figure 16). Despite great elaboration on the drawing, the white blood cells were notably absent.

62

Frequently, patients respond in a less than credible fashion and draw something which indicates to us clinically that probably no real image, or at best a vague image, of the white blood cells has been formed. On the other hand, many patients invest more energy in describing their immune system than any other component of the imagery. The drawing in Figure 9, for example, leaves little doubt that the patient clearly images the white blood cells in a logically consistent fashion. This patient's description of the drawing reminds one of a dramatization, and her mental picture comes across clearly in her description of both the form and interaction of the white blood cells.

Dimension 5: Activity of white blood cells

This scale focuses on the movement of the white blood cells as described by the patient. Frequently, actual dynamics are not discussed or drawn, and judgments need to be based on the capability of, or inherent movement conveyed in, the image. The white blood cells are often described as moving in waves, or as hordes of soldiers marching, or as simply "floating." The first two cases would be given higher ratings since they are clearly more active representations. Another type of discrimination must also be made when rating this dimensions. Activity which is self-generated (as in the case of motion of people or animals or rapidly moving concrete descriptions of white blood cells) should receive slightly higher ratings than activity which is generated external to the image (as in the case of vacuum cleaners or scrub brushes, which were frequently chosen images). The detail described regarding the activity, and the complexity of the activity (providing it is consistent and makes sense), are also factors which should enter into higher scores. The imagery shown in Figure 9 would obviously be considered desirable on this dimension and would, therefore, receive a high score. Drawings containing snowflakes, bubbles, or other symbols which have no energy source of their own, would be scored low. The Activity dimension, together with that of Strength (Scale 9), seem to be important in evaluating the patient's perception of the effectiveness of the onslaught against disease and the nature of the battle, as it were, to maintain or achieve good health.

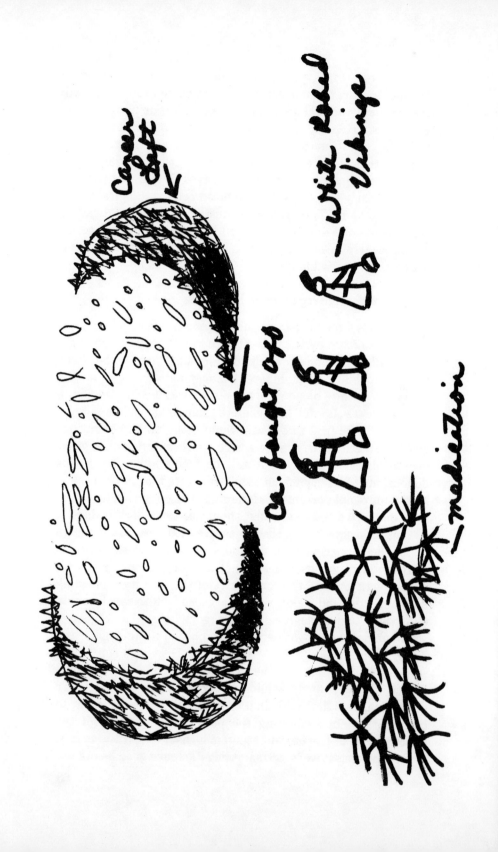

FIGURE 9. IMAGERY RATED HIGH ON VIVIDNESS OF WHITE
BLOOD CELLS (DIMENSION 4)

*The patient described her original visualization of cancer
as a large, pointy, solid mass. The chemotherapy was
described as pills exploding like rockets, covering the
cancerous areas and softening and destroying the cancer
cells. She saw the immune system as countless, white-robed
Vikings with shiny helmets. They carried sharp shovels with
hollow handles that contained a healing fluid. The shovels
are used to chop and pick up the destroyed cancer cells and
then toss them into the blood stream to be carried away.
Then the shovels are turned over and they release healing
fluid from the hollow handles. She says the blackness she
images in her chest is going away, and the tumor is left at
a half-moon shape. The center of her chest looks like Swiss
cheese. She mentioned a spontaneous color change of her
tumor which occurred as she was going through a healing
process. She says she has difficulties picturing her tumors
now and that one has shriveled. She now uses her Vikings
to work on her arthritis, releasing soothing fluid.*

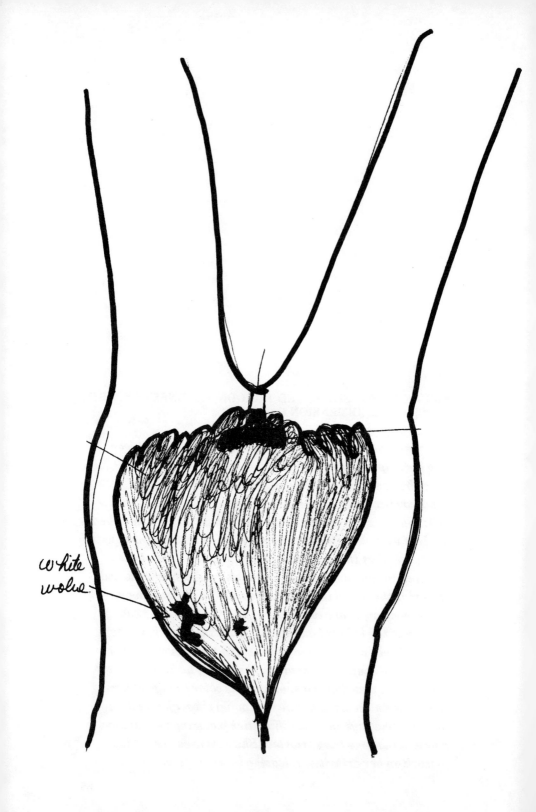

white
wolve

FIGURE 10. SINGLE, DETAILED WHITE BLOOD CELL

The patient describes her treatment only as some pancreatic enzymes which look like hordes of tiny green cells covering her cancer like flies. They gnaw away and fall off when they are full. She occasionally sees them simultaneously with the white blood cells. Both her treatment and white blood cells enter the cancer and eat from the inside out. She has a new image of a tidal wave of blood containing all of her body's resources. It has thousands of white wolves representing her white blood cells. There is an undertow in the wave and that is important as it pulls back with suction and attracts the dead sick cells and takes away the discharge that her cancer is producing. Last week her cancer was pink red and convoluted like a brain. It is full of ligmented, confused cells. Now the wolves get chunks and pieces and it gets smaller. It is confused, and coming apart from the outside in. The wave is very vigorous and full of oxygen. She ends her imagery by seeing the emptiness in her pelvic cavity.

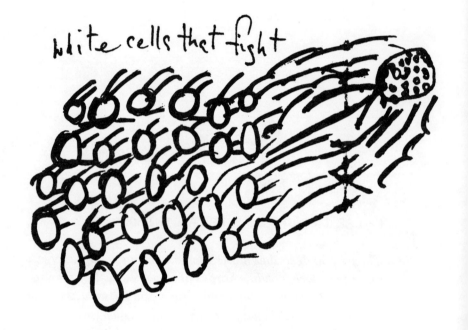
white cells that fight

FIGURE 11. SIMPLISTIC DRAWING OF WBC'S, WITH EMPHASIS
ON NUMBERS

*The patient described her cancer as a small grape. The
grape was more fleshy on the inside, and she could
frequently see them cutting it [during the mastectomy].
It was difficult for her to describe her cancer cells, but
the white blood cells were clear and she described them as
big and strong. She could see them going through to the
cancer cells and trying to invade them. She could see cancer
cells, but only confined to the growth. The growth itself
was described as smaller than the white blood cells. The
white blood cells are round and much larger and stronger
than the cancer cells [4-5 times larger]. She believed that
the white blood cells were strong with the help of the
physicians and God. In her drawing, the arrows represent
the fight that is going on between the white blood cells
and the cancer cells.*

Dimension 6: Numerosity of white blood cells

This dimension refers to the number of white blood cells relative to the cancer cells. The index is based on both the number drawn and the number described. As with the size factor (Scale 7), questions of the patients must be rather pointed such that some actual numbers are given. Patients without any specified instructions will occasionally draw one detailed white blood cell symbol, yet in their verbal offerings will estimate the number in the hundreds or millions. (See Figure 10.) Other instances have been noted where patients will painstakingly draw many, many white blood cells with no details, but are still able to describe the configuration in some complexity. In both instances, high scores should be given on this factor. Low scores are assigned when no numerical information is presented and when the drawing reveals comparatively few white blood cells. Subsequent validation research has shown that Numerosity, like Scale 1 (Vividness of cancer cell), is not as predictive of disease outcome as some of the other factors, yet it has been retained because of the information it contributes to the overall prediction.

Clinically, the inclusion of this factor is quite valuable. Questioning the patient regarding numbers, and later encouraging the belief that there are, indeed, many of these cells, is conducive to the development of the positive attitudes toward disease outcome which enhance the quality of existence. The scale is one of the more laborious to score, in that it requires the synthesis of a great deal of information. However, interrater reliability was high, which indicates reasonably consistent cues are utilized in the judgment.

It was mentioned above that this score itself does not relate significantly to disease outcome. This is probably an artifact of the open-ended instructions, since it is not specified whether the tumor itself or the individual cells should form the basis for the process. Interestingly, the population of patients who did *not* image on a regular basis (Normative Group II) invested more energy in describing or drawing large numbers of WBC, rather than offering details on the form. For example, the imagery in Figure 11 was given a high rating on this factor, and, as is apparent from inspection of the drawing, the imagery is quite simplistic, with sheer numbers being the only outstanding feature.

Dimension 7: Size of white blood cells

The size of the white blood cell as compared to the size of the cancer cell (i.e., the larger the relative size of the white blood cell the higher the rating given) is a fairly obvious judgment when the imager is highly symbolistic. It is sometimes less obvious when patients use more concrete or factual descriptions of the white blood cell. There may also be some confusion if patients choose to visualize their cancer as a solid tumor, with individual cells having little comparative meaning in this case. Questioning of the patient should focus on the issue of relative size so that the point is made as clearly as possible. The high interrater agreement for this scale indicates again that reading between the lines, so to speak, is effective and reliable.

Size is a viable factor in making judgments about patients' attitude toward sickness and health, possibly because the extent to which any drawing covers a page indicates the amount of energy a patient chooses to invest in a demonstration of this sort. Additionally, the size of the drawing may be related to self-concept, as is the case with human figure drawings. Much of what is thought to be true about self appears to be projected into the image of the white blood cell. On a more fundamental level, the size of the white blood cell relative to the cancer cell merely indicates some intuitive probability about the outcome of the disease.

Representative scoring for the case shown in Figure 12 would be high (4). Here, the patient has drawn a white blood cell several times larger than the cancer cell and described the total tumor area as being about 25 times the diameter of a white blood cell.

Dimension 8: Strength of white blood cells

The estimated strength of the white blood cell is one of the most powerful predictors of short-term disease state. Strength implies destructive capabilities of the symbol and the general effectiveness of the immune system in fighting the

71

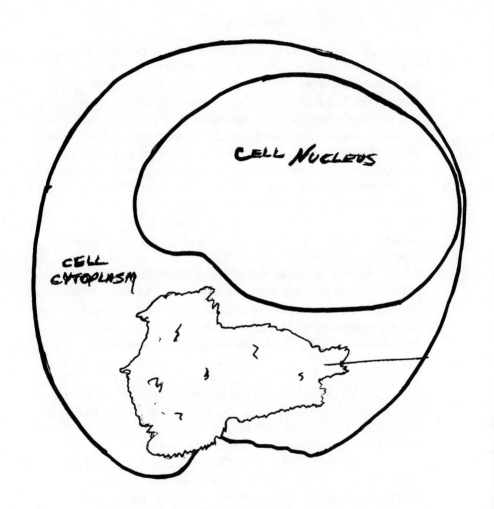

FIGURE 12. IMAGERY SCORED HIGH ON WHITE BLOOD CELL
RELATIVE SIZE FACTOR (DIMENSION 7)

*The patient meditates for 20 minutes and then begins disease
imagery. He acknowledges a creative force within himself
and sees this force operating on various parts of his body
where there may be some abnormality. He sees it in the
thymus, pancreas, adrenal glands, lymph nodes, and nerves.
The cancer itself is described as grey matter, while the
white blood cells look like they are actually dew and
are not seen to him in any symbolic form. He sees the cancer
in different parts of the body. At the time of the drawings,
it appeared to him as large and located in his liver. The
total surface area of the cancer is about 25 times the
diameter of the white blood cells. He sees the attack as
white blood cells tearing up the cancer and engulfing
portions with pseudopods. He said occasionally his cancer
feels like concrete and it is necessary in his imagery to
bring people into this with hammers and chisels. The white
blood cells end with the process of surveillance. He says to
him it is not the quantity of cancer that he sees that is
important, but the amount of time it takes during his
meditation to clear it out.*

73

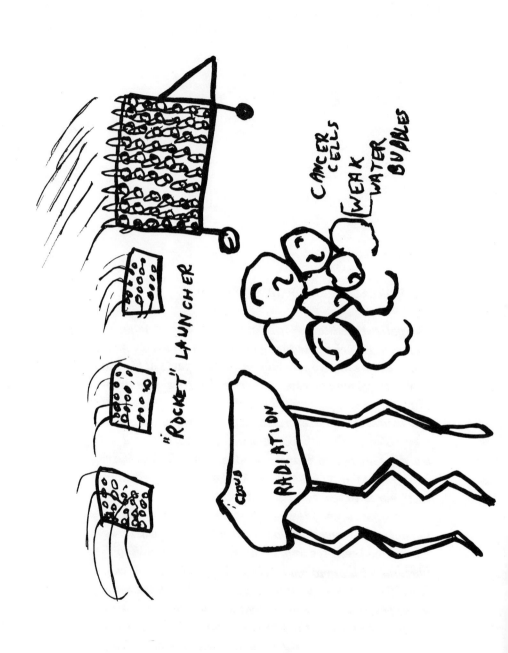

FIGURE 13. POWERFUL IMAGE OF WHITE BLOOD CELL (HIGH
SCORE ON DIMENSION 8)

The patient says he sees a violent attack on his cancer,
like a blitzkrieg. He has a rocket launcher with 50 cylinders.
These represent the white blood cells. He reloads them as
the bone marrow regenerates the new cells. All day he
sees continuous action. His cancer looks like water bubbles,
weak and stupid. There is no space where he used to
picture his cancer. They burst as soon as the rockets
touch them. He says he sees cancer cells blowing up through
normal body processes. His radiation, when he was taking
it, was described as an electrical storm, making water into
steam, and the sweat eliminated the cancer.

disease. The composite judgment on this dimension includes not only the size and inherent strength in the symbol itself, but most importantly, the nature of the interaction of the white blood cells and the cancer cells. Given a particular description, which body of cells is most likely to win what the majority of patients see as a battle in every sense of the word? The nature of the aggression tells us much about whether the patient sees himself as a hapless, passive victim of circumstances, or whether an attempt is being made to psychologically garner resources and defy the cellular proliferation.

Patients view their struggle in a number of qualitatively different and intriguing ways. Frequently, a frenzied attack (tearing, biting, ripping) is described, especially when animals are chosen as symbols. Other patients describe a consistently successful, but more contemplative attack, often with some ritualistic type of movement. The latter cases are usually characterized by deliberation, the former by anger. Both instances would normally be given high ratings, but we assume that the differences are highly representative of other behavior patterns peculiar to the individual patients.

An important cue used to make judgments on this factor is the consistency with which the patient acknowledges the WBC as the winner of the encounter, or as successful in attempts to engulf, dissolve, or otherwise destroy the cancer cell. Many patients express doubt about the totality of the success of the WBC, saying, "Some of the time they win," or "Most of the time they are successful." Generally, when patients see the WBC as losing the fight, especially when they invest some time in describing this event, low scores are given. For example, a "1" or very negative score was given to a patient who described her white blood cells not only as stationary, but also as being attacked and eaten up by the lobster which seemed to symbolize her pain and her cancer cells together. Low ratings should also be given on this dimension when no interaction between the WBC and cancer is described, even though the representations of the cells might be present. Conversely, the "continuous blitzkrieg" action described in Figure 13 was rated high. In this case the cancer cells were weak, stupid water bubbles being attacked by rockets.

THE TREATMENT

Dimension 9: Vividness of treatment

The clarity and conciseness of the treatment being administered is one of the most readily scorable dimensions of the IMAGE-CA. The reason for this, perhaps, is that the description of treatment is usually given with more emotionality, and with the use of more subjectively charged adjectives, than most of the other factors. Patients either seem to regard their treatment as a bane—making them sick rather than well, or are gloriously pleased—attributing it to their disease management. A valuable criteria for judgment is whether or not the description appears well integrated and logical, at least in consistency. When descriptions appear fragmented or when it is hard to follow the train of thought of the patient, low scores should be given. "Treatment," incidentally, is usually defined as surgery, radiation, or chemotherapy. However, many patients choose to discuss nutritional therapy, vitamin therapy, biofeedback, and physical therapy.

There are cases in which cancer patients will not be under medical treatment of any kind, or will not indicate any symbolism for treatment components. The standardization sample had approximately 25% patients with no current medical treatment. Therefore, in order to utilize the formula for weighting and combining all the scales, the evaluator should score persons not on medical treatment as a "3" merely because this figure is the average of all patients and will not add statistical prediction in either direction. However, in order to compare across patients, the scale is necessary for inclusion.

Patients who simply choose not to consider treatment as a viable factor in overcoming disease would be given a "1." Interestingly, it was occasionally omitted altogether from the drawings, despite instructions to the contrary. One of the most vivid descriptions of chemotherapy appears in Figure 14. This patient's output contains an elaborate description of the treatment procedure.

77

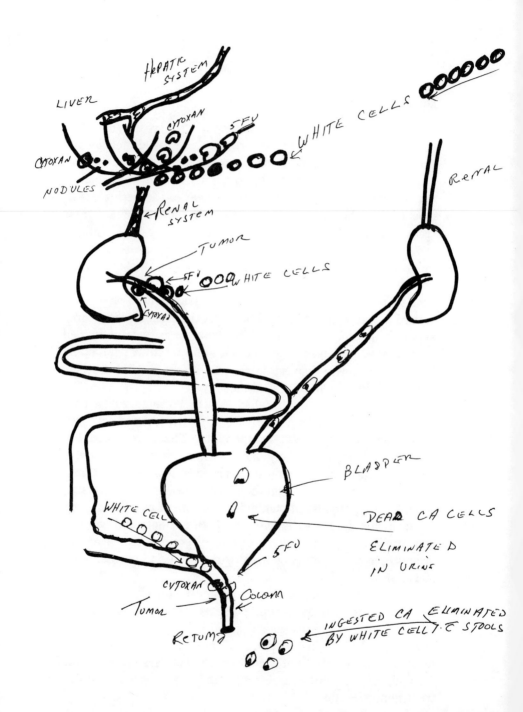

FIGURE 14. VIVID AND COMPLEX DRAWING OF CHEMO-
THERAPY

*The patient describes cancer at each of three sites: [1]
cancer in the liver resembles a black, dot-like nodule;
[2] cancer in the kidney is a velvety braided mass, and
[3] that of the colon is flat and has a smooth finish. It is
black in this instance and always has fewer nodules. He
sees his medication, his cytoxin and 5FU working
synergistically, potentiating one another. The 5FU and
cytoxin have pinchers going into the renal system,
attacking the braided cancer by invasion. Each braid has
one key cell which, when invaded, will allow the whole
thing to let go. It unravels and heals. The white blood cells
are very firm cells with hollow centers that do a cleaning-up
process by ingesting the debris. The chemotherapy generally
is absorbed by the cancer cells or is accepted into the
cancer cells and destroys them from within. He sees
millions of white blood cells.*

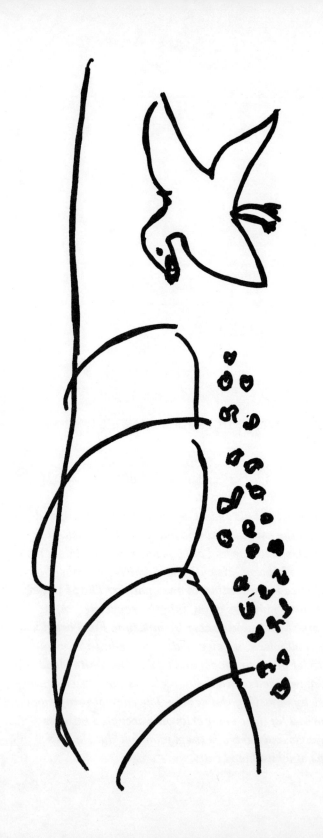

FIGURE 15. IMAGERY RATED LOW ON EFFECTIVENESS OF
TREATMENT (DIMENSION 10)

The patient described in detail two types of white blood
cells — waves and breakers which roll over the sand and
expose and dig up the sand crabs which are the cancer.
The sea gulls [the second type] then grab up the sand
crabs. The patient is basically asymptomatic and has
been for some time. She imaged the described scene,
but could not imagine it being in her body. She always
saw the same number of crabs even after the waves
had washed over them. She could visualize her immuno-
therapy going into her body, but had some revulsion
about it and did not see it doing anything.

Dimension 10: Effectiveness of treatment

The degree to which the patient images the treatment as capable of combating disease. On both Scales 9 and 10 there was high interrater reliability on scoring since descriptions are fairly obvious in this respect. Factors such as the amount of space and time allotted to this description enter into the scoring. The identical assumption is also made for this dimension as the previous one. As with the previous scale, if no treatment is indicated simply score this dimension "3."

An example of an imagery rated low in effectiveness is presented in Figure 15. The patient was quite adamant and detailed about the effectiveness of the WBC, yet felt revulsion when describing immunotherapy—unable to see it doing anything.

GENERAL CHARACTERISTICS OF THE IMAGERY

Dimension 11: Symbolism

This dimension is based on the *degree* of symbolism elected by the patient in describing the disease and healing process. Whether the patient shows a symbolistic interpretation of the cancer, the white blood cells, and the treatments, or a more factual depiction based on some anatomical knowledge may not be predictive of actual disease state in the short run. But, because focusing on this aspect contributes to the effectiveness of the scoring system, it is included in the analysis. It is of some interest that the amount of exposure to anatomical facts does not determine what type of imagery— symbolistical or factual—that the patient shows. It is very common to find that patients use symbolism to represent the cancer cells, but describe the white blood cells as a biologically correct process. This may well have to do with some need to disguise the tumor itself. A mixed type of imagery would be given a "3," while a completely symbolistic imagery would be given a "5."

The type of symbolism selected deserves separate evaluation, since many of the symbols are recognized in the literature on mythology and archetypes, and many patients envision ancient moralistic battles being fought within their body. Factors that have been found to relate to symbolism are discussed throughout this text, but particularly in the sections on psychodiagnostic correlations and the imagery process, and in the case studies.

Dimension 12: Overall strength of imagery

This dimension is dealt with in part in virtually all of the other scales, since it focuses on the patients' overall ability to image. It is a subjective judgment, of course, but is derived from the amount of intensity or emotional investment that a patient seems to give to the percept. As such, the examiner bases considerations on the elaboration of details in the dialogue, the degree to which the person can explain action of the symbols, and the assuredness that a patient imparts that the symbols have actually been experienced and not merely concocted to please the examiner. It is not surprising that this dimension correlates highly with the Betts Questionnaire on Mental Imagery (Betts, 1909)—a measure of perceived vividness of imagery. This factor relates to how *well* a patient seems to be able to image, and not *what* the images consist of. Judgments on the relationship between overall imagery and disease are not included here, but are reserved for Dimension 14.

Dimension 13: Estimated regularity of imagery

As part of the dialogue, the patients are asked to relate how many times a day they participated in the imagery procedure or how frequently they thought about their disease. As is the case with all such verbal reports, it requires consideration in view of the socially desirable aspects of the situation. Not having another independent measure of frequency, the patients' statements were given credibility. It should be pointed out that for Normative Group II (medical school patients), denial of disease anxiety, and hence frequency of thought, seem to be the desirable mode, whereas

with the patients who were using an imagery form of psychotherapy (Normative Group I), frequency of imagery was
desirable. Nevertheless, high scores were related positively
to the overall scoring system in both cases.

Dimension 14: Clinical judgment

This scale is the most complex, yet potentially the
most powerful of all. It requires an integration of the total
reported imagery process, together with a knowledge of
psychodynamics and an understanding of the emotional
aspects of cancer. Primarily, it requires the sensitivity that
comes with experience in working with cancer patients. It is
an opportunity for the evaluator to use all the subtle cues
imparted by the patient that indicate the patient's ability and
willingness to participate in disease management. For naive
judges, high variability is to be expected.

This dimension is largely a scale on which the clinician
can interject his own expertise and experience into the
protocol. The scoring of the previous dimensions can be done
on the basis of objective criteria and little increase in prediction can be gained. However, the clinician should be able to
pick up cues, perhaps unconscious ones, to illuminate the richness of a response. For example, the following characteristics
have been noted as possible predictors of positive health, but
no statistical validation can be formulated since so few cases
share commonalities:

(a) Those cases that have a continuity of symbolism
appear to be strong in imagery. That is, symbols that can be
thought of as being in context with each other and integrated
into a single percept are positive signs.

(b) Those symbols that have a high degree of emotional value attached to them are important in prediction. For
example, if a person has always been afraid of being overwhelmed by bugs, and uses these ideas in their drawings,
their impact has a greater importance than if such characters
were spontaneous.

(c) The more the person appears to maintain the
symbol as a continuous source of comfort or support, the more
favorable the report. For example, the symbol or concept can

84

be utilized as a reference, such as "My watchdogs are usually looking after me," or "My body warriors are at watch *always.*"

SCORING PROCEDURES

In order to determine a patient's overall score, the examiner must combine the ratings of each of the 14 dimensions in three basic steps: (1) transformation of raw ratings (RR) into weighted scores (WS); (2) the summation of the WS (Sum WS); and (3) the transformation of the Sum (WS) to the overall standard score (STEN). The IMAGE-CA scoring sheet provides space for these computations.

The transformation of raw ratings (RR) to weighted scores (WS) is done in order to maximize the relative predictive values for each dimension. There are some dimensions that have greater importance in degree of disease process prediction than others. For example, Dimension 1 (Vividness of cancer cell) has equal importance in prediction as Dimension 2 (perceived activity), and both receive equal weights of unity. However, Dimension 3 (perceived strength of cancer) is empirically more important in the overall scoring and is weighted as being three times the raw rating. The relative weights for each dimension are presented below.

Dimension	1	2	3	4	5	6	7	8	9	10	11	12	13	14
Weight	1	1	3	3	4	1	3	4	2	3	1	6	1	16

In order to transform the raw ratings to weighted scores, multiply each rating by its respective weight. For example, the WS for a RR of 3 for Dimension 4 would be 9 (i.e., 3 x 3), and a WS for Dimension 14 with an RR of 3 would be 48 (i.e., 16 x 3).

The Sum (WS) is simply the arithmetic sum of the 14 weighted scores (WS). For example, the scores listed below for Patient A yield a Sum (WS) of 102, and the Sum (WS) for Patient B would be 202.

85

	Patient A		Patient B	
Dimension	**RR**	**WS**	**RR**	**WS**
1	3	3	3	3
2	3	3	4	4
3	1	3	4	12
4	1	3	3	9
5	2	8	4	16
6	3	3	4	4
7	4	12	3	9
8	5	20	5	20
9	1	2	4	8
10	1	3	4	12
11	2	2	3	3
12	1	6	3	18
13	2	2	4	4
14	2	32	5	80
Sum (WS)		102		202

In order to depict the meaning of the total scores in relation to an overall distribution, the Sum (WS) is converted into standard scores ranging from 1 to 10 (STENS). The conversion is made by locating in Table 2 below a particular Sum (WS) in the left column and then reading directly across to find the associated STEN score.

For the examiner who does not have a table to consult, or the researcher who wishes to convert to more specific STENS, the formula for conversion is:

$$\text{STEN} = \frac{(\text{Sum (WS)} - 170)}{17} + 5.5 \, .$$

When only 13 dimensions are evaluated, the sten scale shown in Table 3 should be used. The exact conversion formula in this case is:

$$\text{STEN} = \frac{(\text{Sum (WS)} - 120)}{9.5} + 5.5 \, .$$

Table 2

CONVERSION OF SUMMED WEIGHTED SCORES TO STENS USING ALL 14 DIMENSIONS

Sum (WS)	STEN
247 or greater	10
229-246	9
213-228	8
195-212	7
178-194	6
161-177	5
144-160	4
127-143	3
110-126	2
less than 109	1

Table 3

CONVERSION OF SUMMED WEIGHTED SCORES TO STENS USING 13 DIMENSIONS

Sum (WS)	STEN
165 or greater	10
153-162	9
144-152	8
134-143	7
125-133	6
115-124	5
106-114	4
96-105	3
87-95	2
less than 86	1

Missing or Nonapplicable Ratings

There are times when some dimensions are either inappropriate or missing. For example, there are some patients who are not in treatment, or not taking their medication; therefore, Dimensions 9 (Clarity of treatment) and 10 (Effectiveness of treatment) are unscorable. Also, Dimension 14 (Clinical evaluation) becomes an extremely important criterion as the examiner gains experience. However, while the initial cases may be learning cases, the 14th dimension may be eliminated altogether. The scoring system should, in these instances, be based only upon the first 13 dimensions and their respective weights. Table 3 should be used for sten conversion.

Meaning of the STEN

The intent of any scoring system is to make one record of responses comparable to another. However, it is mandatory that the clinician keep in mind that the usefulness of this instrument may be justified on a broader perspective than "a score." For example, the content and descriptive terminology may be of greater assistance in facilitating communication between doctor and patient, or greater understanding within the patient, than a quantifiable status. Moreover, the dynamic understanding of relating to another person's concerns about their disease is the goal of this technique, and the score is merely a method of condensing the dimensions to one continuum.

With precaution of clinical consideration, the STEN score is descriptive of the sample characteristic from which the technique was normalized, and indicative of predictive prognosis. A person's sten score, presented in STENS, will range from 1 to 10, with respect to a normal distribution with a mean of 5.5 and a standard deviation of 2.0. In terms of variance, this means that patients with scores in the range of 5-6 are in the average range. Scores in the ranges of 3-4 or 7-8 are slightly below or above average. Scores in the 9-10 or 1-2 ranges are considered significantly different from the average response.

88

1, 2	3, 4	5, 6	7, 8	9, 10
extremely lower	slightly lower	average	slightly higher	extremely higher

In terms of prediction, the meaning of the total STEN is more general and is based on patients' disease process. To facilitate interpretation, the score categories are best divided into three disease processes. Validation research (to be considered in detail later) indicated that patients who received a STEN of 3 or less displayed rapid physical deterioration and died of their cancer in the two-month follow-up. Patients who scored in the 4-7 range had average stability, and those who scored 8 or greater showed remission or significant decrease in tumor size.

To be more precise in score discrimination is not possible at this point in the development of the technique. Perhaps the variances within these categories reflect the degree of judgment on the clinical dimension.

1, 2, 3, 4	5, 6	7, 8, 9, 10
poor prognosis	expected prognosis	excellent prognosis

III

CASE STUDIES

It is only when dealing with the qualitative portion of the imagery work that we become aware of the extent to which the imagery process is integrated into every facet of the patients' existence: their disease status, their behavioral repertoire, their personality traits. The struggle against death is an awesome battle, for which strategies are developed as a result of lifelong experiences and competencies. In order to demonstrate the relationships between symbols and disease, the richness of the cognitive effort, the extent of the mental involvement in the course of malignancy, portions of case histories are presented. An ever-present task for us is to identify threads of commonality among outstanding patients.

SYMBOLS AS SYMPTOMS

The place or the medium of realization is neither mind nor matter, but that intermediate realm of subtle reality which can be adequately expressed only by the symbol. The symbol is neither abstract nor concrete, neither rational nor irrational, neither real nor unreal, it is always both. . . .

C. G. Jung
Psychology and Alchemy

Just as the body exhibits symptoms which are not the disease itself but unique manifestations of the interaction of the disease with the total body, the psyche does likewise. In the case of the latter, however, symbols become the synthetic representations of the more concrete cognitive processing. The analogy between symbol and symptom can be carried into application, in that the understanding of both symptomatic and symbolic events lead to the diagnosis of a patient's physical functioning and psychological attributes. In essence, we are dealing with the same process. Physically, certain clusters of symptoms have been analyzed over time to the extent that they are rather consistent harbingers of known physical disorders. From a clinical standpoint, the choice of symbolism seems to be likewise appropriate for taxonomy, at least to the extent that various symbols can be related to stabilization or remission, whereas others seem to be associated with physically downhill process.

The use of visualization or imagery in diagnostics is unusual in the scientific sense because, although it is generalized to physical events, the protocol unfolds from a unique level of the personality. The symbolism most commonly relates to a person's framework of what symbols best relate to his or her perceived psychological attributes of the disease process. These symbols are derived from a combination of resources, including memory, dreams, and visions. Many of the symbols identified are ancient archetypal figures; many are traditional representations for figures of good and evil.

The symbols of positive connotation are those representing strength and purity; powerful enough to subdue an enemy—pure enough to do so with justification. Such images frequently take the form of knights or they may appear as Vikings—heroes only slightly removed in time and place from the white knights. The knight is an archaic symbol from fairy tales to which most of us have a common exposure. It is interesting that patients form other associations with the white knight, including the description of their activities which highly resemble a soap commercial from a few years back. Most importantly, patients who use this imagery typically respond favorably in the treatment process.

Other frequently used symbols which appear to be positive predictors of favorable disease process are those of large, powerful animals, especially dogs and bears. These are usually good symbols associated with a healthy attitude.

94

However, it should be pointed out that it is the competencies that the animal displays in the drama that identify the real meaning of the symbol for the patient. For example, one patient saw bears as his immunological system and snakes representing cancer cells. Sometimes the snakes attacked the bears, and the bears did not have enough strength to fight back, according to his dialogue. So, regardless of the inherent properties of this symbol, the competency was muted. Even though the suggestion is frequently made to patients in a therapeutic situation that they adopt animal imagery, some of them refused, finding it repulsive to see an animal tearing apart a living thing. One patient who had a very weak imagery was instructed to imagine her cancer as raw meat and the white blood cells as polar bears; but she reported it was extremely nauseating to her because of the blood and violence. We feel that a supreme amount of violence, or particularly gory or vicious imagery, may not be particularly advantageous. It may rob the patient of some energy that he or she could invest into the the healing process rather than into the recapitulation of anger and destruction. From a physiological point of view, this frequent recapitulation associated with emotions of anger may be extremely detrimental to the patient's health, especially when there is not an avenue for positively dealing with negative feelings.

Patients with an overall "good" imagery rarely describe mechanical devices, such as vacuum cleaners, automatic sprinklers, shovels, or picks, that might be used to dig out the cancer. A few patients describe only a pair of hands tearing out the cancer or performing some other type of destruction. In no case was this imagery ever associated with a favorable turn in disease. There are many speculations as to whether these symbols characterize a detachment the patient may feel toward his bodily processes or whether they relate to other personality characteristics. Our current feeling is that the symbols are negative in part because they do not have a natural source of energy of their own and hence the patient may feel limited or dependent. Highly destructive elements such as fire, poisons, and acids are not generally described by patients who are doing well. These symbols apparently relate to the degree of discomfort and pain experienced.

95

In regard to the predictive aspects of imagery, the symbol of ants is a particularly poor sign. It is typically selected by women (never, in fact, has it been used by a male to our knowledge), and it has been used to identify both the white blood cells and cancer cells. Case after case has demonstrated a positive correlation between disease increase and this sign. One psychological interpretation is that ants produce a regenerative trail that is virtually impossible to eradicate. Although one or two ants could be destroyed, it may be impossible to completely defend against this symbol. Crustacean creatures such as crabs, scorpions, lobsters, or even octopi—animals that have in common a tentacle (or a claw) that clings or grabs—are not good symbols from a statistically predictive standpoint. It is not surprising that the word "cancer" is derived from the Latin word for crab, the traditional association being based on a similarity of physical resemblance between the legs of a crab and the growing tumor.

The majority of unhealthy patients tend to be symbolistic in describing the disease element, while the white blood cells are seen as more concrete. The patients with the poorest prognoses spent much more energy symbolizing the cancer cells, perhaps as a way of masking their horror and anxiety associated with the disease. The patients with more favorable prognoses usually reflect more investment of energy in their projections of immunological mechanisms.

Examiners should place emphasis on the content of imagery, since the symbols selected very often are representative of personality traits in the patients. It is important to consider the symbols in context, in the dynamic sense of their projection. One must be cognizant of the existential struggle the patient is attempting to describe. The extent to which the patient can express this enterprise in a meaningful form depends on the person's creativity, background, and personal ability at a given time to convey his feelings in verbal or nonverbal symbols.

THE PATIENTS

Negative Images

A beautiful young woman with breast cancer that had spread to her lungs and clavicle drew the very anatomical pictures shown in Figure 16. She was able to visualize the radiation machine shooting at the cancer cells, the cancer cells trapped in a bulging clavicle, and the chemotherapy in her bloodstream. She was unable to describe or draw anything relating to her white blood cell activity, nor did she picture any interaction taking place between the chemotherapy and the abnormal cells. After 4 days of intensive therapy geared toward attitude change, she was still unable to give a coherent picture of these activities. Her human figure drawing (Figure 17), according to just about anyone's criteria, shows a lack of self-identity. She was, incidentally, trained as an artist. She had experienced two most unsatisfactory relationships with men, very much desired a long-term relationship, but felt she didn't have the energy to begin again. She returned home and died within a few weeks, although according to her physician, "She shouldn't have." Her lesions themselves were minute, and she had been strong and physically active.

A young man with metastatic melanoma was unable to visualize any activity taking place between his white blood cells and his cancer (See Figure 18). The cancer cells appeared as happy clown faces, and the white blood cells as tiny dots. He said that the dots occasionally flirted with the cancer cells, but were never able to attack. During the course of therapy, the patient was able to reduce his Demerol intake by about 75%, but continued to experience new tumor growth.

Animals in Action

Not only is the interaction between cancer cells and white blood cells of some significance, but also the relative strengths and weaknesses of the white blood cells and cancer cells as represented in the imagery. A 14-year-old girl who was diagnosed with cancer of the liver described her white blood cells as large dogs and her cancer cells as slugs (Figure

97

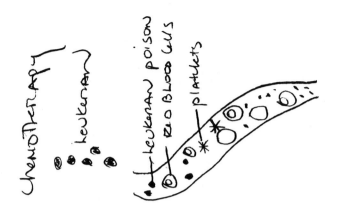

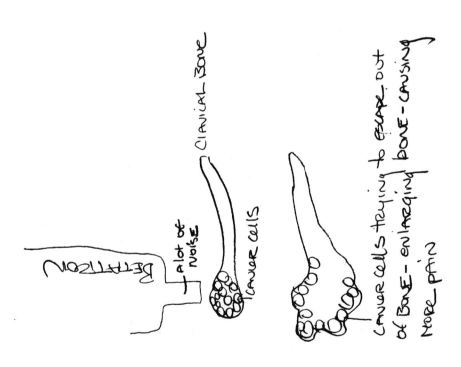

FIGURE 16. ANATOMICAL DRAWING WITH OMISSION
OF WHITE BLOOD CELLS

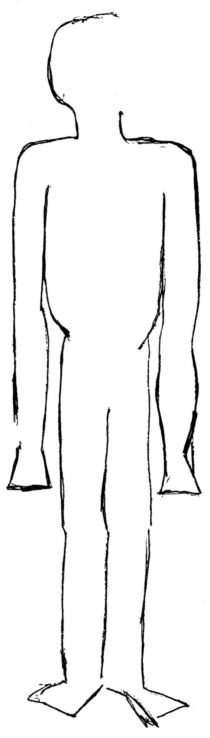

FIGURE 17. HUMAN FIGURE DRAWING BY A YOUNG ARTIST

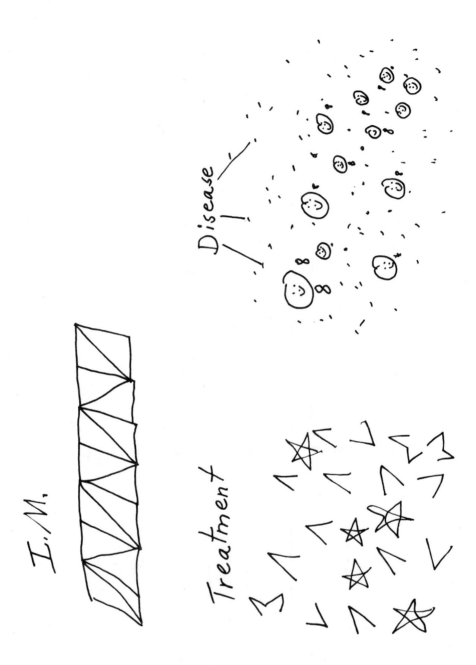

FIGURE 18. CANCER CELLS AS CLOWN FACES

19). She saw her liver as red and perfect except for one dime-sized spot. She described many dogs in her imagery, and they all enjoyed eating the slugs. She has experienced a superb turnaround in her disease, and, according to the last medical report, she is disease-free. It was mentioned previously that many of the patients who do well use large animals to represent their white blood cells, and that while big animals are regarded as "good" imagery, ants or small insects have not been related to good disease management. Figure 20 shows the imagery of a 28-year-old woman with metastatic liver cancer who used the symbol to depict both her cancer and white blood cells. The patient, a lovely, gentle woman and mother of two young children, died within weeks after the drawing was made. Ants—scourge of the homemaker—leave the unending trail which eventually defies the exterminator. This particular patient was virtually identical to several other women in the sample in terms of diagnosis, type of the treatment, previous health history, and age. From our perspective, the single differing characteristic appeared to be in attitude as expressed in the imagery analysis.

Many patients describe their cancer as the traditional crab. As we discussed in the section analyzing content, crabs or crablike creatures are not generally associated with good disease outcome. One breast cancer patient from our indigent population produced the drawing in Figure 21. She visualized her cancer as a red lobster running down her right arm. White blood cells were seen coming from the rest of the body, but were eaten up by the lobster. The lobster was described as moving slowly, with claws coming out.

White Knights

One particular symbol crops up over and over: The white knight as a representation of the immune system. Perhaps it reflects exposure to soap commercials, or maybe to a more basic impression that dates back to the hero on a white horse. This symbol has been observed by other therapists in similar work and in our recent studies with medical school patients. Another beautiful example was drawn by a gifted woman, one of the few who has had minimal disease (cervical

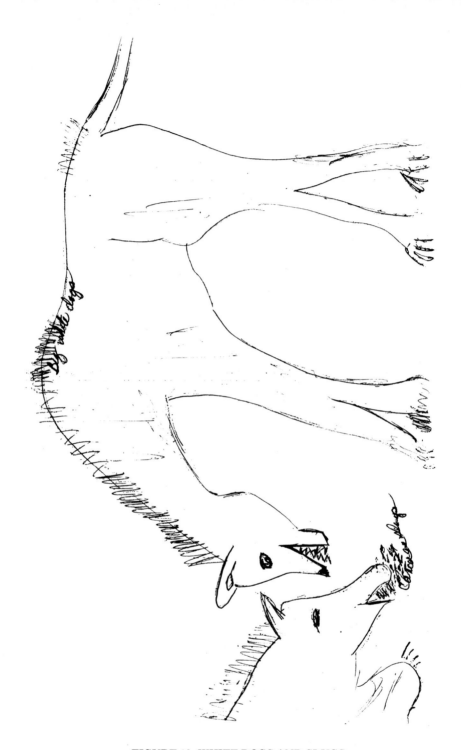

FIGURE 19. WHITE DOGS AND SLUGS

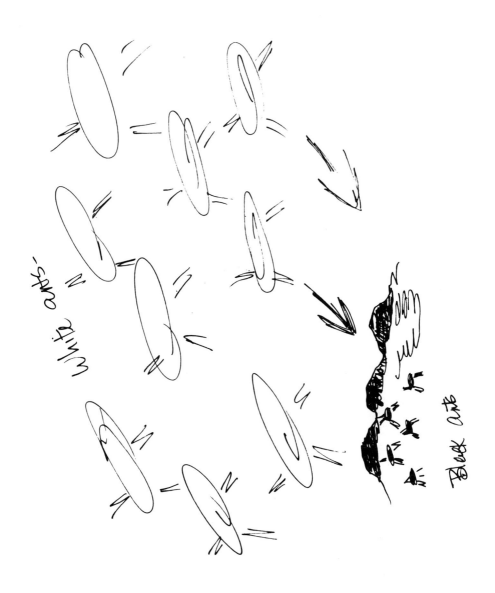

FIGURE 20. WHITE ANTS AND BLACK ANTS

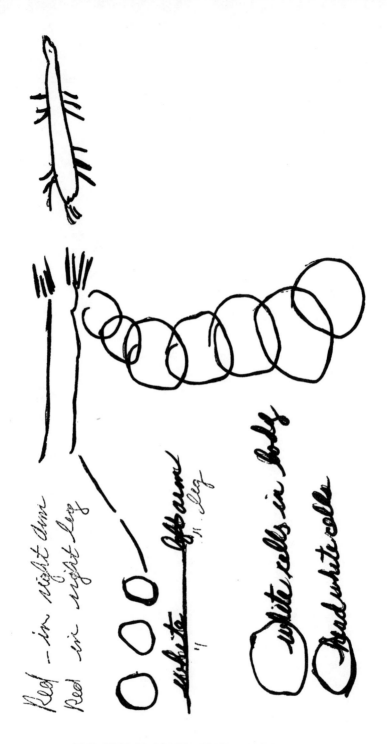

FIGURE 21. CANCER AS A LOBSTER

cancer) and who chose the therapy as a means of preventing recurrence (Figure 22). Support for the consistency of this image across populations was obtained in our interview of a breast cancer patient being treated at the county hospital. She described her white blood cells as armies of knights, attacking the cancer cells with swords. They wore white robes with a cross on the front, "sort of like Sir Richard." Her drawing (Figure 23) is primitive, but her dialogue was virtually identical to the private patients we examined. She had no previous imagery training, per se, and only one exposure to the IMAGE-CA Relaxation and Guided Imagery tape.

The symbol was also used by one of the most unusual patients we have had the opportunity to study. He is a physicist diagnosed over a year before testing with cancer of the pancreas which had spread to other areas. The prognosis for this type of disease is grim, regardless of medical treatment. His imagery deserves a special treatment (See Figure 24). He initially described his cancer cells as armadillos, and his white blood cells as white knights (Figure 25 represents a detailed drawing). The knights had a daily quota (he works for the major organization whose byword is "quota") of creatures they needed to spear on their lancets. They were then wiped off in the bloodstream which contained the chemotherapeutic agent. At one time during his therapy he observed that many of his white knights were dropping or disappearing. He was subsequently informed that his white blood cell count was dropping. Fearing that he would be taken off chemotherapy, he was determined to "peg" the number of white blood cells. After making this decision, the white blood count stabilized, and the chemotherapy continued. Sometime later, he experienced some difficulty in the white knights meeting their daily quota. They were beating the bushes to find the armadillos. Shortly after, he underwent ultrasound diagnosis and there was no evidence of tumor. One of the major problems that he is now confronting in his imagery is a lack of spontaneity. To overcome this, at the conclusion of his meditation he envisions a little boy shaking hands with an adult (Figure 26). During one difficult period recently, he regularly saw the boy on roller skates, gliding by most unobtainably. This very unusual patient seems to be in touch with his

105

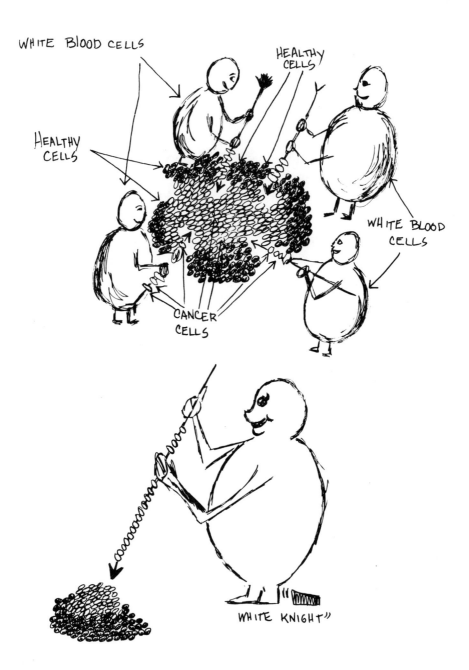

WHITE BLOOD CELLS

HEALTHY CELLS

HEALTHY CELLS

WHITE BLOOD CELLS

CANCER CELLS

WHITE KNIGHT"

⬤⬤⬤⬤⬤ NORMAL HEALTHY CELLS
OOOOOO CANCER CELLS

FIGURE 22. WHITE KNIGHTS

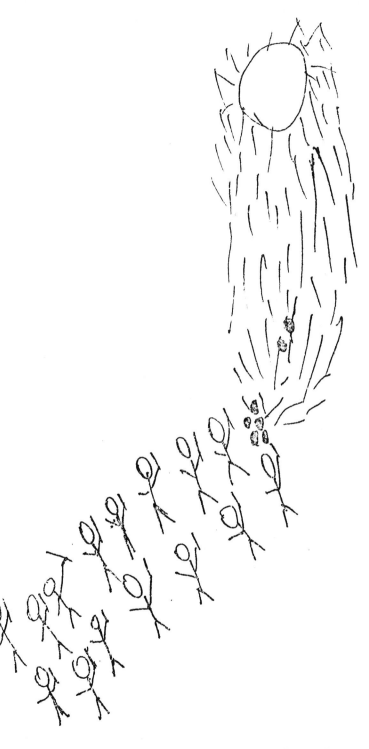

FIGURE 23. "SORT OF LIKE SIR RICHARD"

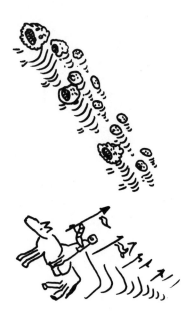
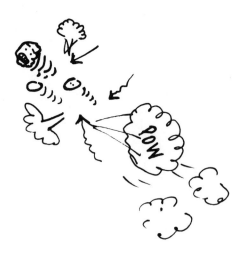

FIGURE 24. WHITE KNIGHTS AND ARMADILLOS

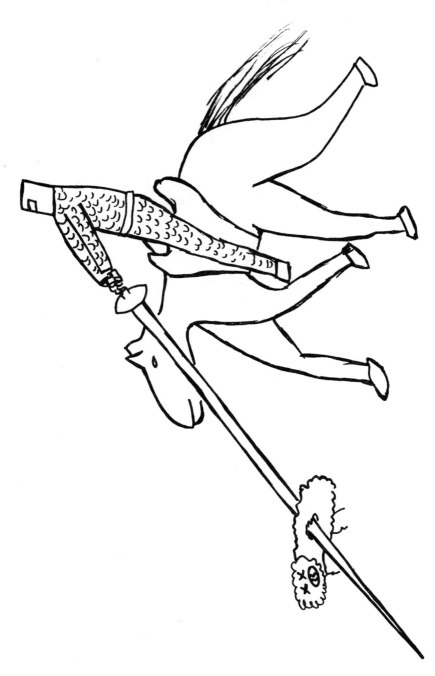

FIGURE 25. DETAILED DRAWING OF WHITE KNIGHT
STABBING ARMADILLO

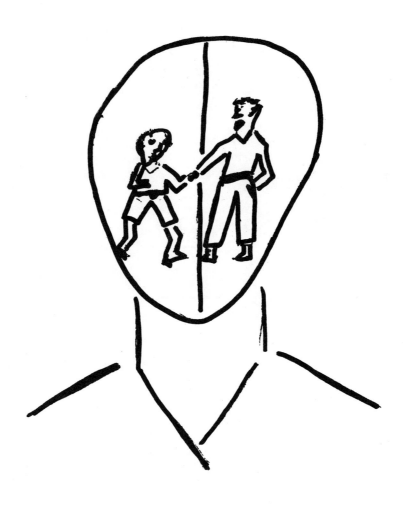

FIGURE 26. IMAGERY BEYOND DISEASE

emotions, and most in control of the expression of them. Perhaps he is similarly in touch with, and in control of, his physical processes.

Realists vs. Symbolists

The physicist's drawings are highly symbolic in spite of his knowledge of cell activity. The basis of choice of symbolic versus actual representations remains somewhat of a mystery and appears to have only a moderate relationship with disease state and to educational background. Most patients try on both types of images and settle on one that feels right to them—occasionally apologizing for the seemingly fictional nature of their choice. The imagery in Figure 27 was produced by a woman with advanced lymphosarcoma. She is a clinical psychologist whose disease has been fairly stable over the last year. Her imagery, likewise, has remained unchanged except for an increasing clarity in description and detail in drawings (Figure 28). Much of the imagery of the white blood cell is quite accurate in terms of what is known about phagocytic activity, cellular membrane permeability, and cellular histology.

Treatment Side Effects

The majority of patients examined were receiving either chemotherapy or immunotherapy. The former acts on the principle of any poison or cellular toxin. The cancer cells, which are weak and metabolically confused, are more likely to be destroyed. The healthy tissue is affected to a lesser degree, since the cells' reparative processes are intact. The chemotherapy, therefore, is accompanied by a multitude of side effects produced by its toxic effect on the system. The side effects vary greatly from patient to patient, in some cases being debilitating, and in others, almost indiscernible. They include nausea, vomiting, digestive upsets, hair loss, and blood count changes, to mention a few. The variance can be attributed to the type of chemotherapeutic agent and the general physical condition of the patient. There is also

111

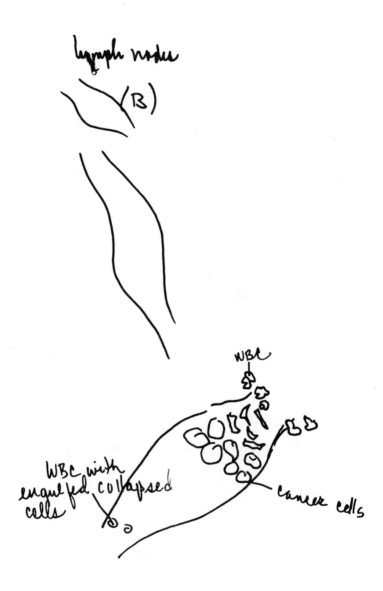

FIGURE 27. ANATOMICAL IMAGERY OF LYMPH NODE

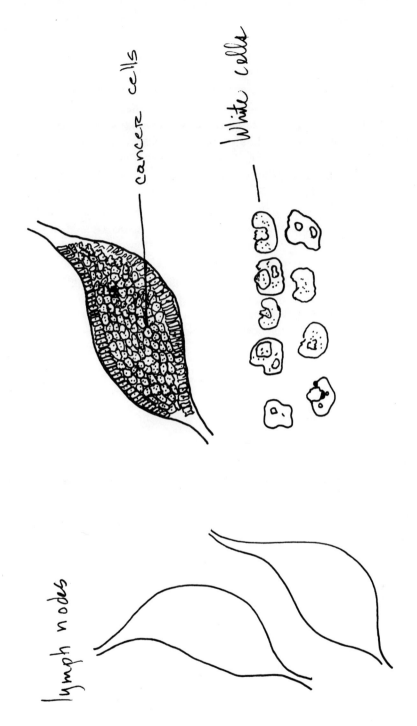

FIGURE 28. DRAWING OF NODES WITH INCREASING CLARITY

probably a lot of expectancy thrown in for good measure. One patient who was receiving an injection every 2 weeks had pronounced side effects the week following therapy, and then was free from the effects until the day of his next injection, at which time he reported having stomach cramps, nausea, and so forth, prior to administration of the drug. That is difficult to account for by any rebound effect of the drug. The role of expectancy (what a patient "expects" to happen as a result of the treatment) can be studied by examining the patients' descriptions of their images of the chemotherapeutic activity. One of the patients, a woman with primary breast cancer which spread to the liver, remained robust physically and did not even experience the hair loss that usually accompanies her type of treatment. She described her chemotherapy as acting like soy sauce. It was sucked up by the cancer (she used the analogy of the way the liquid is soaked up by a napkin), and the cancer cells were described as shrinking and shriveling. She described it as running off the pink, healthy tissue much like soy sauce runs off bean sprouts (Figure 29).

Sensory Modalities for Imaging

Apparently, there are a lot of ways to skin the cat. All of the patients seem to use visual imagery, either exclusively or in part. Some seem to be more adept at auditory imagery. In particular, two musicians favored the auditory mode. They would talk through the imagery rather than form mental pictures, which seems a reasonable thing for a musician to do since the favored or trained sensory modality is auditory. One of the musicians was diagnosed with an 8 cm lesion in his brain. Prior to radiation, he was aphasic, unable to string two words together. His wife persistently began to involve him in imaging his disease. She talked through the meditation with him, she drew pictures on the back of his hand (using the tactile sense which is notably resistant in the face of even massive brain damage), and found pictures in magazines for him to look at to help in visualization. The initial picture that he drew of his disease was a circle. Within 3 months, he offered us a two-page, beautifully phrased description of his meditation.

114

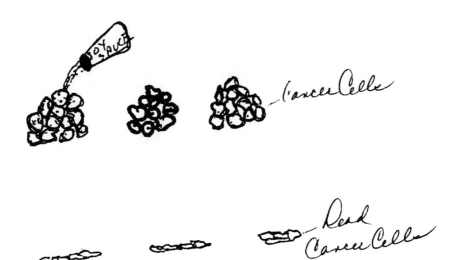

FIGURE 29. CHEMOTHERAPY AS SOY SAUCE

Persistence of Images

Working with a patient to alter imagery so that it reflects a more positive expectancy is frequently readily accomplished. At other times it is a task fraught with trauma and difficulty. In such cases, the reasons underlying the resistance require sensitive investigation. For example, a 73-year-old gentleman with widespread head and neck cancer produced the drawing in Figure 30. The white blood cells are represented by snow flakes falling down on his shoulders. He said he could see no other interaction between the white blood cells and cancer cells, simply that they were "drifting down." Sensing our dissatisfaction with his drawing, he produced a second drawing during his lunch hour which is presented in Figure 31. The differences between the drawings are simply that one has arms and hands and the other does not. Perhaps self-image improved, but certainly the dynamics of his cancer imagery remained unchanged. His tumors continued to grow and he died within a few weeks after presenting the drawings. He remained active until just before his death, continuing to enjoy golf, hunting, and fishing. Pain for him was a rarely experienced phenomena. When questioned about this, he replied that he had devised an imaginary bulldog which would chomp up any painful twinges that he noted. It was suggested many times during the course of a week that he use a symbol similar to the bulldog to represent his white blood cells. He replied, "No, I don't think I could do that. The bulldogs are too powerful." Irrational, perhaps. But on the other hand, dying a painless death at age 73, reflecting upon a good life, and continuing activities which one loves most is a rather envious position. Any attempts at intervention or convincing the patient to fight to alter the course of the disease may be highly disrespectful of a patient's inner desires.

Surveillance or Monitoring of Imagery

Patients who systematically image their disease process frequently undertake a unique form of surveillance imagery when symptoms abate. The drawing in Figure 32 is an example produced by a woman with metastatic breast

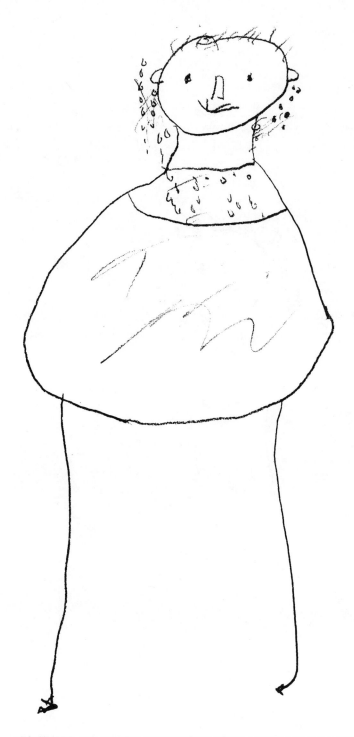

FIGURE 30. EXAMPLE OF INEFFECTIVE WHITE BLOOD CELLS

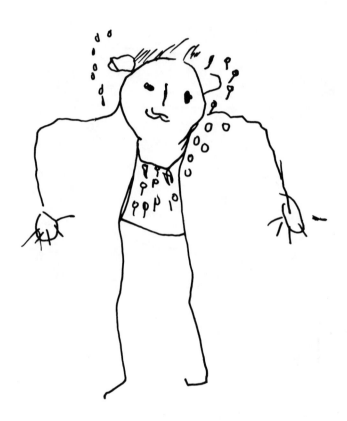

FIGURE 31. DUPLICATE DRAWING AFTER COACHING

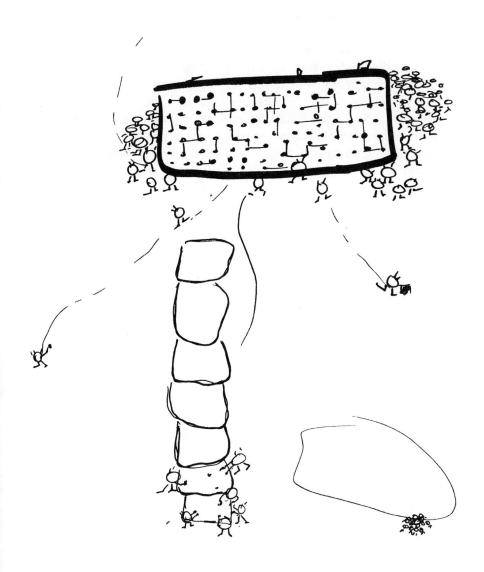

FIGURE 32. CANCER SURVEILLANCE

cancer who, at the time of the drawing, had no evidence of disease according to a bone scan. She had continued an active professional life with only slight interruption during treatment. She envisioned her white blood cells as miniature doctors who, being alerted by a switchboard, travel out into her bloodstream to destroy any abnormal cell that appears. Like many patients, she utilized her disease in a positive way. She gained new and valuable insights into life and it was enriched accordingly. Whatever else the surveillance imagery does, it most certainly gives patients a feeling of involvement in returning to health and, hence, a feeling of being less victimized by any physical setback. It also keeps patients conscious of and in touch with their body's processes.

IV

STANDARDIZATION AND RESEARCH WITH THE TECHNIQUE

$\mathbb{T}$he section related to the reliability and validity of the technique is actually a series of researches involved with these issues. In reality, there is no such thing as one validity coefficient for a psychological construct. Rather, the researcher has to correlate the measure with a variety of meaningful constructs in order to articulate the definition of the instrument.

Two normalization studies were conducted on two different samples of the cancer population in order to determine the reliability and validity of the technique. An intercorrelation analysis with other psychological and neurophysiological measures is also presented to clarify the meaning of the imagery dimensions.

NORMATIVE STUDY I

The sample on which a test is standardized should represent as closely as possible the population for which the technique is intended. The distribution of demographic variables with respect to the subjects in the standardization sample is presented in Table 4. The 58 subjects of this study had been diagnosed at the time of admittance as having metastasized cancer and approximately a 5% chance of 5-year survival.

It should be pointed out that the distribution was skewed from the general population on the educational attainment variable with a mean of 17 years. Moreover, there also appears to be an overrepresentation in the number of subjects from the western part of the USA. However, this group is

Table 4

DEMOGRAPHIC DATA OF NORM SAMPLE (N = 58)

Age	Representation	Education	
61-	4%	Below High School	1%
51-60	38%	High School	16%
41-50	29%	Some College	25%
31-40	19%	College Graduate	19%
21-30	6%	Post College	48%
-20	4%		

Sex Types		Geographical Regions	
Males	38%	North	50%
Females	62%	South	50%
		East	22%
		West	78%

indicative of the type of individual who was available to this type of testing at the time of technique development. That is, there was a natural selectivity due to limited practice of psychological intervention with cancer patients.

Reliability

The reliability coefficient is designed to describe the degree to which a test is measuring something of substance. In other words, if an instrument was only measuring error variance, there would be no consistency within itself. The reliability of the IMAGE-CA was measured by two methods: (1) interdimensional correlation, and (2) interrater correlation. The intercorrelation matrix of the 14 dimensions is presented in Table 5. The bottom line represents correlations of each dimension with the total score.

If a test is consistent within itself, the dimensions will correlate positively with one another and account for predictive variance in the total score. The correlations presented in Table 5 should be carefully considered by the clinician when analyzing the dimensions separately. The smaller the correlation of a given dimension to the rest of the technique, the less confidence one can have in making inferences concerning the importance of that dimension. For example, Dimension 1, the Vividness of the cancer cells, is less important in the scoring than 12, Overall imagery strength.

Interrater reliability measures the degree to which two or more people perceive the same stimuli independently and rate the dimensions consistently. In this case, two raters scored the protocols without the knowledge of the other's ratings. In fact, one of the raters had absolutely no knowledge of who the patients were or their involvement in the program. The raters had only a record of the interview content and the drawings. The coefficients for each respective dimension are reported in Table 6.

For the observant reader, it should be pointed out that the correlations are all statistically significant, yet have a wide range (.60 - .95). Narrow variances tend to produce lower reliability correlations. This is reflected in the means and standard deviations shown in Table 7.

125

Table 5

INTERCORRELATION MATRIX OF THE 14 DIMENSIONS

	1	2	3	4	5	6	7	8	9	10	11	12	13	14
1	—	.14	−.12	.43	.13	−.17	.13	.18	.23	.24	.22	.30	.06	.09
2		—	.20	.09	.19	.05	.11	.11	.20	.24	−.05	.32	.07	.23
3			—	.09	.32	.34	.19	.42	.25	.26	.06	.51	.17	.42
4				—	.49	.09	.53	.44	.26	.32	.42	.61	.32	.46
5					—	.16	.49	.51	.21	.24	.29	.62	.32	.49
6						—	.11	.12	.03	.09	−.11	.19	.16	.14
7							—	.42	.26	.34	.15	.46	.25	.38
8								—	.13	.13	.17	.61	.20	.46
9									—	.63	−.02	.37	.23	.25
10										—	.16	.49	.28	.48
11											—	.23	−.10	.22
12												—	.35	.79
13													—	.29
14														—
Total Score	.27	.30	.55	.67	.70	.22	.58	.67	.44	.60	.31	.93	.40	.86

Table 6

INTERRATER RELIABILITIES (N = 58)

Scale I	.63	VIII	.79
II	.74	IX	.95
III	.60	X	.87
IV	.82	XI	.87
V	.82	XII	.73
VI	.77	XIII	.84
VII	.73	XIV	.78

Table 7

MEANS AND STANDARD DEVIATIONS OF DIMENSIONS
(N = 58)

Dimension	Mean	Standard Deviation
1	3.82	.84
2	3.47	.71
3	3.40	.90
4	3.88	.82
5	4.00	.79
6	3.64	.83
7	3.66	.71
8	3.67	.90
9	3.34	.85
10	3.24	1.00
11	3.43	1.38
12	3.35	1.00
13	4.05	.89
14	3.00	1.17

The measurements were analyzed as to commensurate levels, not only to compare consistency but also to determine whether the judges were in agreement as to absolute levels. The Agreement Coefficient (Lawlis & Lu, 1972) was computed using as criterion an agreement of judgments within one interval (K = 1). The results yielded a significant concordance (Chi^2 = 607.23, p < .0001), which suggests virtually 100% agreement.

Validity

In consonance with the theory that the only unambiguous way to define constructs is to demonstrate a correlation to external criteria, the combined dimensions were utilized to predict concurrent physiological health status and a 2-month follow-up of health status. In this study health status was based on objective medical criteria: death, evidence of new tumor growth and degenerative disease, stabilized condition, evidence of reduction in existing tumor(s) and positive process, and evidence of complete absence of tumor(s) or disease. Decisions regarding health status were made independent of the scoring of the IMAGE-CA.

Two separate regression analyses were computed. The first analysis utilized 13 dimensions, omitting the clinical judgment scale (Dimension 14). This analysis allowed the researchers to estimate the power of prediction on the basis of primary objective data, similar to the power of prediction of a novice evaluator. Multiple regressions were also computer analyzed utilizing the clinical experience dimension. The validity coefficients for both analyses are presented in Table 8.

The comparison between the two R coefficients for the 2-month follow-up reveals a very important outcome. Even though both predictions were highly significant, the impact of clinical experience is reflected in a 25% better variance coefficient. Therefore, two separate cutoff distributions were derived.

Tables 9 and 10 contain the weights which are assigned to each dimension according to its relative importance to the overall scale. For a novice scorer (one with less than 50 supervised administrations and scorings), the 14th

129

Table 8

VALIDITY COEFFICIENTS (Regression)

	R	R adj.
Concurrent Disease Process		
with clinical judgment	.76	.71
Two-month follow-up		
without clinical judgment	.53	.50
with clinical judgment	.78	.76

Table 9

CRITICAL CUTOFF SCORES WITHOUT CLINICAL JUDGMENT
(for novices)

Variable	Weights	Total Score	
1	1		
2	1	Mean = 119.38	
3	3	S.D. = 19.01	
4	3	140 or above =	50% patients show no
5	4		evidence of disease
6	1	=	70% show diminished or
7	3		no disease
8	4	=	90% show stabilized,
9	2		diminished, or no disease
10	3	120 =	54% show diminished or
11	1		stabilized disease
12	6	=	46% show new growth or death
13	1	100 or below =	100% show new disease
			or death

Table 10

CRITICAL CUTOFF SCORES WITH CLINICAL JUDGMENT

Variable	Weights	Total Score	
1	1	Mean = 169.26	
2	1	S.D. = 34.25	
3	3		
4	3	198 or above =	43% of patients show
5	4		no disease
6	1	=	93% of patients show
7	3		regression of tumors
8	4		or no disease
9	2		
10	3	150 or below =	100% of patients show
11	1		new cancer disease
12	6		or died
13	1		
14	16		

dimension should be omitted and the weights in Table 9 should be used. More experienced clinicians should refer to Table 10.

After multiplying each score by its weight, the resultant products are summed for a total score. If Table 9 is used and the score is 140 or above, the prognosis is excellent for the diminishment of disease. If the score is less than 100, the prognosis is poor. No prediction can be made for scores between 100 and 140. If the clinical opinion can be computed (the highest weight of all the dimensions), much more powerful predictions are possible. Using the weights in Table 10, 93% prediction was obtained for favorable prognosis and 100% for unfavorable (198 - 150). Again, the range between 150 and 198 is uncertain.

Statistical analyses are exactly that, statistical. Consequently, the numbers do not reflect the intuition so extremely helpful in determining the individual's investment in his own health. The fact that a person's score might be 98 does not condemn him to an early grave, just because a sample of similar individuals justifies such a prediction. The clinician is encouraged to use the statistical description merely to provide a frame of reference for his decisions, not to serve as his decisions.

NORMATIVE STUDY II [1]

The second validation study for IMAGE-CA substantiated two aspects of the previous results: (1) the reliability of interjudge dimensions, and (2) the concurrent validity of the IMAGE-CA with disease process. However, a more dramatic strategy was to demonstrate that the IMAGE-CA reliability and validity coefficients held up for a sample of cancer patients of a lower socioeconomic level.

The sample of 21 cancer patients treated in a medical school-affiliated county hospital were administered the IMAGE-CA in the standardized form. The demographic data for this sample is presented in Table 11.

---

[1]The work upon which these data were gathered was performed pursuant to Contract 1-CN-45133 with the National Cancer Institute, Department of Health, Education and Welfare, as part of the patient evaluation effort.

133

Table 11

DEMOGRAPHIC DATA OF THE LOW-SOCIOECONOMIC GROUP

Percentage of Sample	Educational Level
60%	6th-9th grade
25%	4th-6th grade
15%	less than 4th grade (were omitted from analysis)

All subjects were residents of Dallas County with income less than $3,000 annually.

Reliability

Since the purpose of this validation study was to substantiate the findings of the initial work, a broader range of judges was employed. Three judges scored each protocol independently, without the knowledge of other ratings and without any information about the patients. The intercorrelations between the ratings were converted to Fisher Zs, averaged, and converted back to correlation coefficients as averaged reliabilities. These coefficients are presented in Table 12. The ratings were subjected to an agreement analysis using the identical criterion (K = 1) as Study I. The results were significant (Chi^2 = 198.02, p < .0001), indicating 95% agreement.

Validity

The ratings for each dimension were averaged and weighted according to the weights derived in the regression analysis of Study I. In this study, the criteria for concurrent validation were ratings of patient functioning given by the medical school social worker. The particular formula for patient functioning was based on the *Patient Status Form*, a format for listing patient activities. Originally developed by Izsak (1971), the current *Patient Status Form* is an adaptation with more clearly scaled items involving medical and functional rehabilitation areas. A measurement of ability (reliability = .70) is based on the following criteria:

A. General Activity

   Pain
   Nutrition
   Sleep
   Frequency of medical follow-up
   Looking after oneself
   Sexual activity

B. Working Ability

   Attitude toward work
   Work activities

Table 12

AVERAGE RELIABILITIES OF VALIDATION STUDY II

Dimension	
1	.84**
2	.83**
3	.69**
4	.67**
5	.82**
6	.50*
7	.60**
8	.53**
9	.66**
10	.63**
11	.82**
12	.61**
13	.59**
14	.71**

* $p < .025$

** $p < .01$

C. Social Adjustment

Relationship to physician
Relationship to partner
Relationship to children
Relationship to relatives

The *Patient Status Form* is a 14-item questionnaire utilizing a four-level assessment on each of the functional entities, ranging from 3 (no limitation) to 0 (no functionability). The items were summed and divided by the total appropriate for the disease. The resultant overall scores ranged from zero (no function in any area) to 1.00 (fully functional in all entities).

The results of this concurrent validity analysis revealed significant convergence between the IMAGE-CA and the *Patient Status Form* with consideration of Clinical judgment (Dimension 14) held constant ($r = .45$, p $< .025$). Clinical judgment was withheld since, for the most part, the researchers had very little clinical interaction with this particular patient sample. Also, after looking over the protocols, it appeared that the low-socioeconomic-level sample was somewhat different than earlier ones (middle class) with regard to achievement, self-concept, and attraction. When the Clinical judgment was added to the variance of the IMAGE-CA, the validity coefficient remained significant ($r = .37$, p $< .03$) but reduced in predictive variance. In other words, the researchers were correct in assuming negligible ability to predict clinical progress with this group, since the prediction actually added error to the relationship.

A regression analysis was performed to compare the weightings of the 14 dimensions of this study to the weightings in the previous study. The multiple R when adjusted for sample size was .47, very little different from the .44 of the previous weighting system. When the beta weights were compared to the standardization sample, only Dimensions 1 and 14 were relatively different. Dimension 1 (Vividness of cancer cells) had a moderate negative loading instead of a low positive one, and Dimension 14 (Overall clinical judgment) had a moderate positive loading instead of a very high one.

137

Summary

The second validation study did substantiate the first study in major respects. It must be remembered, however, that it was not a replication or cross validation. Neither similar subjects nor similar criterion were utilized. White, middle-class, highly educated cancer patients with Stage IV disease having some background for imagery were administered the technique in the initial formulation. In this second study, low-income, mostly indigent, and racially mixed patients were used. Many of the patients in the latter group were considered primarily postsurgery mastectomy patients whose disease process varied from "no known disease" through widespread metastasis.

Cultural differences were evident in the administration of the instrument. Very little urgency was noted in the second sample, as if their cancer problems were only a small part of their overall lot in life. There were only a few complaints about their future and a tremendous amount of acquiescence. In contrast, the first or higher socioeconomic group seemed to regard the diagnosis as a far greater disaster and were actively seeking out new and promising treatments.

The criterion for the initial group was degree of tumor involvement, whereas, the criterion for the second group was degree of functionality. The choice of criteria was evidently the major concern of each group at this time in their lives. It was noted that the second group did not have a long-term follow-up, an unfortunate consideration since that was the variable that was so predictable in the first study.

The ratings for the studies were made by people trained in psychology and social work with graduate degrees. Specific training in imagery analysis required approximately 50 hours, including administration, scoring, and clinical practice. Competency with the technique probably does not require graduate training per se, but basic interviewing skills and human sensitivities are critical to valid results.

IMAGERY VARIABLES AND PSYCHODIAGNOSTIC RELATIONSHIPS

In order to determine whether the individual dimensions on the IMAGE-CA were related in any way to psychological functioning of the patients, correlations between these items and subscales on a battery of psychodiagnostics were determined (N = 101). The tests used in the study included the Minnesota Multiphasic Personality Inventory (Hathaway & McKinley, 1942), Levenson's Modification of the Locus of Control (Levenson, 1972) which yields three subscales— Internal, Powerful others, and Chance, The Firo-B (Shutz, 1967), and the Profile of Mood States (POMS). Virtually all of the dimensions on the IMAGE-CA related in an understandable fashion to various subscales on the diagnostics. Those variables that were significant are presented in Table 13. The most interesting aspect of the study was the finding that, by and large, the items that involved imaging the cancer were related primarily to scales which could be classified as "Trait" scales, i.e., seem to be reflective of the more permanent and enduring characteristics of the patients. On the other hand, factors related to the imaging of the white blood cells involved a preponderance of mood "State" characteristics. Thus, these data suggest that white blood cell imaging would be highly variable and highly dependent upon current factors, whereas cancer imaging would be the more endemic to the patient. It should also be pointed out that cancer imaging did not relate to short-term disease progress to the extent that the white blood cell factors did.

In light of these data, perhaps we need to reconsider the current thrust to understand the premorbid personality characteristics of the cancer patient, and begin to focus more concisely on postdiagnostic psychological response. This is very much in line with our view toward the psychophysiological mechanism involved in the psyche-soma interaction during cancer process. That is, mood directly affects and interacts with immunological enhancement or deficiencies. Attitude toward treatment, as reflected by the imagery Dimensions 9 and 10, seem to be a mixture of state and trait characteristics, as do the last four items involving the more generalized

139

Table 13

IMAGERY VARIABLES AND PSYCHODIAGNOSTIC RELATIONSHIPS
(N = 101)

Imagery Variables	r^*	Psychodiagnostic Variables
Cancer		
Dimension 1 - Vividness	.37	Firo B - Wanted inclusion
Dimension 2 - Activity	.20	POMS Confusion
	—.35	Locus of Control Powerful Others
	—.26	Locus of Control Chance
	—.40	Firo B - Wanted Inclusion
Dimension 3 - Strength	—.31	Locus of Control Chance
	—.30	MMPI - scale 1
	—.37	MMPI - scale 7
	—.36	MMPI - scale 8
	—.24	POMS Depression
White Blood Cells		
Dimension 4 - Vividness	—.29	MMPI - scale 5
	.28	Firo B - Wanted Affection
	—.34	MMPI - F scale
	—.26	POMS Tension
	—.24	POMS Depression
	—.29	POMS Anxiety
	—.23	POMS Confusion
Dimension 5 - Activity	—.26	MMPI - F scale
	—.22	POMS Tension
Dimension 6 - Numerosity	—.29	MMPI - scale 4
Dimension 7 - Size	—.23	POMS Anxiety
Dimension 8 - Strength	—.20	POMS Anxiety
	—.34	MMPI - F scale
	—.26	Firo B - Expressed Inclusion
	—.27	POMS Tension
	—.26	POMS Depression
Treatment		
Dimension 9 - Vividness	—.25	POMS Anxiety
Dimension 10 - Effectiveness	—.27	Locus of Control Powerful Others
	—.21	POMS Anxiety
	—.30	MMPI - scale 5
General		
Dimension 11 - Symbolism	—.20	POMS Fatigue
	—.22	POMS Confusion
	—.38	MMPI - Control
	.54	Firo B - Wanted Affection
	—.31	POMS Depression
	—.37	POMS Anxiety
Dimension 12 - Overall Strength of Imagery	—.33	MMPI - scale 5
	—.28	MMPI - scale 8
	—.34	Locus of Control Chance
	—.26	MMPI - scale 2
	—.24	POMS Depression
	—.27	POMS Anxiety
Dimension 13 - Regularity of Imaging	—.29	MMPI - F scale
	—.27	MMPI - scale 7
	.31	Locus of Control Internal
	—.27	POMS Tension
	—.26	POMS Depression
	—.29	POMS Confusion
Dimension 14 - Imagery and Disease Management	—.26	MMPI - scale 1
	—.30	Firo B - Expressed Inclusion
	.30	Firo B - Wanted Control

$^*p < .05$

gestalt of the imagery process. A more complete discussion and interpretation of the dimensions follows.

CORRELATIONS OF THE INDIVIDUAL DIMENSIONS WITH PSYCHODIAGNOSTIC VARIABLES

Dimension 1: Vividness of cancer cells

The solitary item correlated with Vividness of cancer cells was the Firo-B scale, Wanted Inclusion. It appears that this scale basically reflects the psychological characteristic of needing to be part of social groups, perhaps requiring social approval, and, indeed, some fear of solitude. This scale is generally perplexing because, even though it seems vital to the imaging process itself, it does not correlate with rehabilitation variables, disease variables, nor apparently with psychological characteristics.

Dimension 2: Activity of cancer cells

The patients who saw their tumors as less active (and hence received higher scores) were more confused, gave moderate or little attribution to external control factors, and expressed a tendency to be very self-sufficient. The overall psychological description seems to impart some degree of internal strength. If this belief is of long standing, then a mood of prevailing confusion is quite understandable. Cellular proliferation or cells out of control are not consistent with the psychological dimensions in this category.

Dimension 3: Strength of cancer cells

The weaker a patient imaged the cancer cells (and hence the higher score), the less belief that chance was a factor of control. Basically, however, the scale seems to reflect both depression and anxiety: the less anxious, less depressed patients apparently envision the cancer cells as weaker, while the more depressed and anxious patients describe their cancer cells as relatively more overbearing.

141

Dimension 4: Vividness of white blood cells

As mentioned above, in this analysis the white blood cell dimensions related primarily to the mood state scales. Among the significant correlations, tension, depression, anxiety, and confusion were all determined by the Profile of Mood States. This seems to indicate that the more vivid a patient's imagery, the less expression of the basic negative state. Additionally, the patients who score high on this dimension typically seem to be quite honest and express vocational and avocational interests which are homotypical.

Dimension 5: Activity of white blood cells

Patients who describe their white blood cells as being quite active seem to be rather open, honest, and relatively less tense. This dimension seems to reflect little in the way of psychological characteristics, yet was found to be highly predictive of current follow-up disease and rehabilitation status.

Dimension 6: Numerosity of white blood cells.

The single scale on the psychodiagnostic battery which correlated significantly with the number of white blood cells described by the patient was MMPI Scale 4 which in a normal population probably describes conformity vs. non-conformity. The more white blood cells relative to cancer cells the patient described, the more conforming according to the MMPI scale. Thus, a social desirability factor in reporting numbers may be operative in this case.

Dimension 7: Size of white blood cells.

The relative size of the white blood cell described by the patient appeared in this study to be related only to state anxiety. The less anxious the patient, the larger the relative size of the white blood cell described.

Dimension 8: Strength of white blood cells

As with Dimension 7, low state anxiety seemed to be related to the positive attribution of strength to the white

142

blood cell. Other state characteristics, such as low tension and lack of depression, were similarly related. Patients who respond in a fashion indicative of self-sufficiency also identified more strength in their white blood cells. The MMPI F scale, a validity index, is also predictive of this dimension. Based on an interpretation of this scale, one can conclude that patients who comprehend the task, are cooperative, and who do not seem to be disorganized by severe anxiety states generally score high on white blood cell variables.

Dimension 9: Vividness of treatment

The clearer and more comprehensively a patient is able to relate the *modus operandi* of the treatment, the less state anxiety exhibited on the psychodiagnostic instruments. This was the only factor found to statistically relate to this dimension. Again, we point out that highly anxious patients obtain low scores on many of the dimensions of the IMAGE-CA. Effective imagery seems to have all the characteristics of a successful desensitization process.

Dimension 10: Effectiveness of treatment

Patients who described their treatment in a way that appears to be more effective generally had less expressed belief in the external control of powerful other people as manipulators in their lives and were more likely to exhibit interests typical of the same sex. Anxiety, again, was negatively correlated with this dimension of strength of treatment.

Dimension 11: Symbolism of treatment

The more symbolistic the patient's imaging process, the less momentary fatigue and confusion, depression, and anxiety he exhibited. Patients high on this dimension also expressed needing more affection and attention, and could possibly be identified as somewhat lacking in self-control. To be quite colloquial, patients who feel "good," and yet seem to require some type of nurturance typically use more symbolistic imagery. The process appears to be related to

143

these factors and totally unrelated to either rehabilitation or disease status.

Dimension 12: Overall strength of imagery

Patients who score high on this item, reflecting how well the evaluator thinks the patient is able to image, are less depressed and anxious, more coherent and less confused, and more sex-typed than patients who appear to be weak imagers. Chance also seems to be given little emphasis as a ruling ingredient in the determination of their lives.

Dimension 13: Regularity of imagery

Based on these results, patients who participate in a highly regular process of guided imagery are also less tense, less depressed, and less confused. They are also internally controlled individuals who exhibit some orderliness, or perhaps even rigidity and meticulousness.

Dimension 14: Relationship to disease management

Patients who were judged to have subsequent good disease management based on their overall imagery are typically less depressed, require less social interaction with other people, and are more passive in the sense of acknowledging a willingness to advocate control or management of various factors in their lives. While this appears somewhat anomalous, it makes sense when one considers that the patients who score high on this item may be expressing a willingness or desire to have their disease controlled.

NEUROPHYSIOLOGICAL CORRELATES OF IMAGERY

Few individuals lack the ability to evoke images. However, there is considerable variance in the degree of clarity and vividness of images, and presumably concomitant differences in neurological functioning during the process. Therefore, it seemed to be important to relate imagery to the autonomic experiences of the individual in some fashion. The original research, conducted by Ms. Donna Kelly-Powell, investigated imagery from a selected group of cancer patients for whom visualization or the imagery process was a significant part of the method of treatment they were receiving for their disease and whose data were included in Normative Group I. The first phase of her study was primarily concerned with a comparison of various imagery measures, including EEG recordings, between experienced and inexperienced imagers. In Phase 2 of the study, the EEG measures were compared with the scores on the IMAGE-CA. In addition, ratings on the IMAGE-CA were correlated with pulse rate, a measure of physiological anxiety, and the Betts Questionnaire on Mental Imagery (Betts, 1909).

The results in Phase 1 confirmed the notions suggested by Brown (1974) and others that visual imagery is accompanied by alpha suppression in inexperienced imagers, whereas experienced imagers are able to sustain alpha during imagery. No significant differences were noted on the Betts between experienced and inexperienced groups. The Betts measures an individual's perception of his own ability to image vividly. Since no differences were noted in perceived ability between these two groups of patients, we must seriously question utility of the instrument—since imagery, like most functions, is likely to increase with practice. Self-report on vividness of imagery is probably highly contaminated by the obvious social desirability of certain answers and the subtle and not-so-subtle pressures that patients must feel in a psychotherapeutic milieu that focuses on an imagery procedure. Alpha suppression, then, rather than the Betts, appears to be the most valuable predictor of imagery experience.

The IMAGE-CA dimensions correlated primarily with the stage of imagery during which patients were asked to imagine the process of the cancer cells being attacked. Both Symbolism (Dimension 11) and Overall clinical judgment (Dimension 14) appear to be the primary covariants with the alpha measure. Decreases in alpha during this imaging period appear to be correlated with both increased symbolism and linked with the clinical judgment regarding prognosis. In this

145

particular study, Dimension 12, which is primarily an estimation of patients' ability to image, and the overall prognosis used to determine the judgment on the 14th dimension seemed to be related to the Betts Questionnaire. The pulse rate measures also showed trends toward significant correlations with the symbolism score.

More well-controlled research utilizing exacting features are needed for the alpha level to be fully appreciated and accepted as a correlate of the Vividness of imagery. The significance of the increased or sustained alpha levels for experienced imagers also needs to be considered in other applications.

V

OTHER APPLICATIONS

OF THE TECHNIQUE

The IMAGE-CA is based on the ultimate disease; the most curious and devastating and subsequently the most feared illness of our times. Causes and cures have defied billions of dollars and man hours of the most talented and highly qualified sort. The course of the disease within any given individual is virtually impossible to predict (except within some broad statistical limits)—and even cellular doubling time for any site varies greatly from patient to patient. Yet patients, simply by describing their disease, treatment, and immune system, are able to define their health status with far more accuracy than even blood chemistries (Achterberg, et al., 1977).

The accuracy of the IMAGE-CA and its implications for treatment of cancer have led us to begin a study of other health conditions which are better understood and more amenable to control. Our approach is similar to the cancer study: We have begun by talking extensively to successful or remarkable patients. Virtually all attribute their success in stabilizing or overcoming the condition to some internal process change in self-image, or a conversion of some type which allows them to examine themselves in a new light.

In this section are portions of interviews, pictures, and preliminary data on three of the conditions to which we have applied the IMAGE. A final discussion regarding a special kind of imagery is included—the visions of a spiritual type that give patients prediagnostic information or comfort during the last days of their lives.

149

DIABETES

Scattered reports indicate rather outstanding success using biofeedback techniques with diabetics. As patients learn to relax themselves, insulin requirements have been reported to drop dramatically (Fowler, Budzynski & Vandenbergh, 1976). Encouraged by these reports, we have initiated the development of an IMAGE-D to study the imagery process, relating it if possible to disease outcome.

Diabetes, unlike cancer and the common cold, does not lend itself to such a clear-cut description of a "battle" between an offending presence and an immune system. The biochemical and cellular malfunction, i.e., the inability of glucose to enter cells, is poorly understood, and the purpose of insulin as an aid to allowing the blood glucose to enter cells is difficult to explain. Patients are accustomed to identifying the high levels of blood sugar as the primary culprit—not some mystical (to them) cellular mechanism.

Our developmental efforts have been very much facilitated by our interviews with a 40-year-old diabetic, who was diagnosed when he was 12. Extensive portions of our interviews are included because Dave (not his real name) is the epitome of a successful patient, and has devised a unique imagery process which he uses in combination with an exercise program. He has remarkably controlled symptoms and has decreased his insulin requirement over the years. His drawings appear in Figure 33*a-f*.

Interview With a Successful Diabetic

Dave: I guess all my life I have heard about how bad the disease is. You very seldom see anything good about it. Kidneys go out and you go blind, you get heart disease, it affects your arms, legs, and your potency. I guess I probably lived negatively for a long time myself. Raised a little hell and didn't take care of myself which I don't advocate to anybody. I would like to say also that I am a firm believer that you have to realize that you do have diabetes. You have got to say, "yes, I have got something, something that has to be watched and something that has to be

150

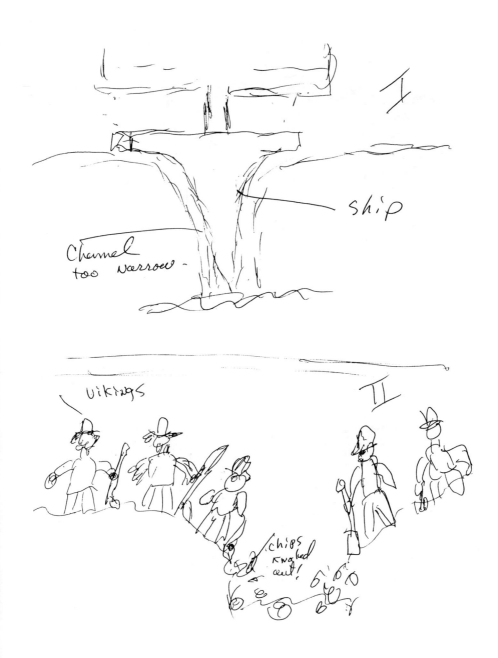

FIGURE 33a. SERIES OF DRAWINGS OF DIABETES IMAGERY

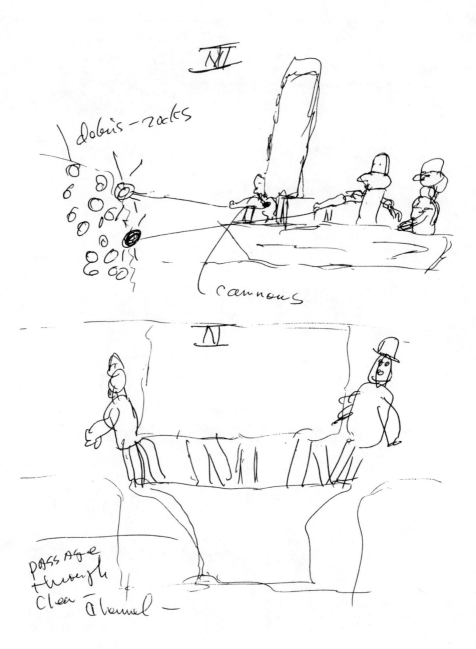

FIGURE 33b

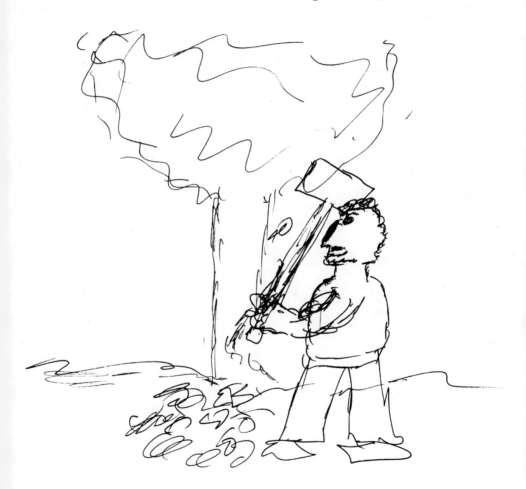

FIGURE 33*c*

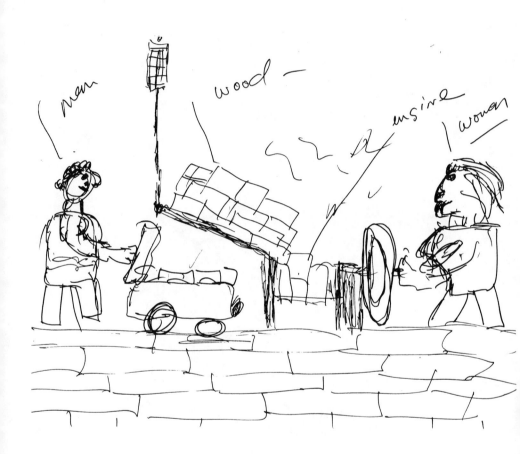

FIGURE 33d

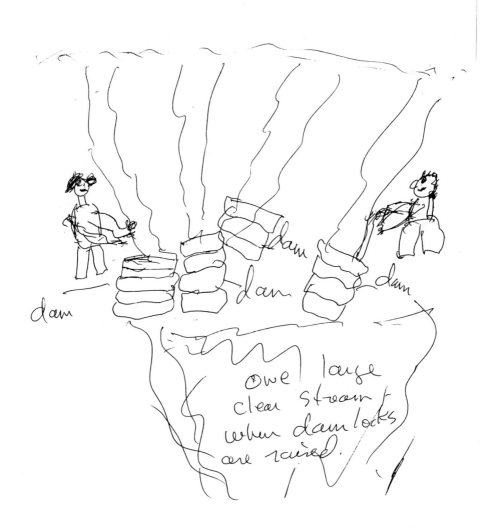

FIGURE 33e

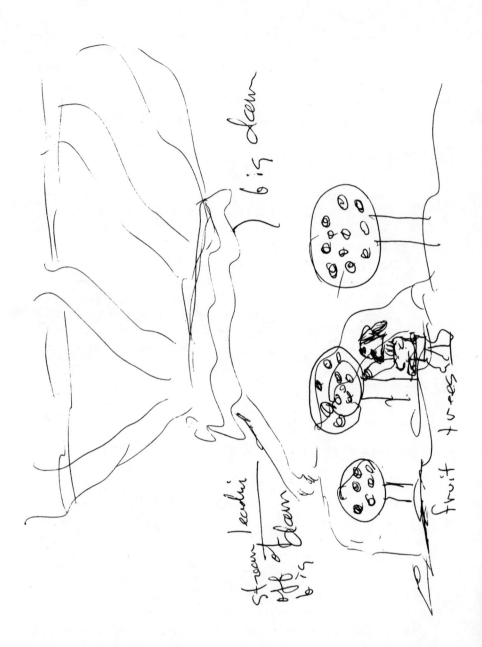

FIGURE 33f

taken care of," but I also think that you can use your mind and use your self to not let the disease cripple you. And that has always been my striving, to try and find something to let me exist with diabetes, realizing I had something that I had to watch but also could lead a very normal life.

Researcher: Were you taking a lot of insulin?

Dave: Yes, I was taking quite a bit. Before I started with imagery and the running that I am doing I was taking 50 units. That's ⅓ more than I take right now. I was always floundering around looking for something to help me with the disease, something. I think I was looking for some things to help counter the bad things that were happening as much as the disease. I got sick of hearing people tell me what I was going to have go wrong with me. "You are a diabetic, my God," you know. I was looking for some way I could deal with that. I got where I really did not like to hear that and I still don't. I think that was another reason I got into imagery and exercise. Like how in the hell could I deal with this negative stuff? I have always been an exercise freak and have known that was good for diabetes. And I have always played tennis or something but I have never really done it day by day like I am doing now. Well, I am jogging about 5-6 miles a day. When I started I was only jogging about half a mile or a mile. When I started running, I was not thinking about the energy or anything. When you run you are burning off so much of the calories, at that time I did not know how many calories you burned off running. One day when I was running I got to thinking about this imagery stuff. I'd done a lot of reading about the mind and how powerful it was.

Researcher: Tell us about your first imagery.

Dave: Right about this time I found out I had the beginning of diabetic retinopathy in my right eye. It was just a tiny hemorrhaging—just beginning. The imagery I used at that time were Vikings in the old Viking ship; and they were in the big fjord rolling down toward a real narrow stream. The only way they could get through was to use their

157

hands and clubs and other tools and chisel these rocks out. Vikings represented my body trying to clear out these blood vessels. The stream was my blood vessels. The rocks were the closing off of the blood flow. I envisioned what would happen the way the vessels in my eyes would shut and would rupture because there would not be any place for the blood to go. I would envision the stream as being narrower and the Viking getting this ship through the channel, and they would be out knocking the rocks down and making a channel for the ships to come on through and, of course, the ships would float on the rushing blood. That is what I was using on my eyes at first because I was so worried about going blind. I went back to the doctor and examined my eyes and they found years later there had been no change in my eye.

Researcher: Do you see any kind of similar image for your blood?

Dave: Well I got to thinking, hell, if I can do it with my eyes, why can't I do it with the rest of me? And so then, I envisioned in my mind a man and a woman. At first it was just a man, strong, built, in great shape, muscles, a little bit like me. He lives on the top of this mountain and there's this tremendous valley stretching down below me. When I started out there was water coming over the mountain, going down to this valley; it was very heavily polluted water. So he wanted to clean up the valley and water, and what he started doing was building a series of dams and then streams. All the time that he is doing this building and chopping the trees down, I think that this is very important for me because he's doing this all by hand. He doesn't have a chain saw to help him, all this is hand work. I envisioned that the docks that he built, and the dams are made out of huge walls that he had latched together himself with rope that he had plaited himself.

Researcher: Okay. What are the dams for?

Dave: They're blocking the stream, to block up enough water to block up the pollution. I should say the pollution is in the valley. Up above the mountain the water is pure. From the top of his mountain it's pure, but down below it's full of pollution.

158

Researcher: What does that mean in terms of your disease? When you see that kind of pollution being in the valley like that?

Dave: I think I see that as maybe potential of what the disease could be, but as long as you fight it, as long as you work at it, it stays pure. Like right now I don't see pollution but what I can see now is a little man raising the gate on this beautiful blue water that is rushing down through the valley. The pollution represents sugar or probably high blood sugar, that is the bad thing. You get high blood sugar and eventually that causes your arteries to choke up. But anyway, since then I have added a woman and she helps with the man. One thing I do about my pancreas is to try and vision my pancreas as this giant. I said I don't have any mechanical things but this is my pancreas as a giant steam engine. What they fire this thing with is wood that they go out and chop down by hand. And they will go up and will build this thing, kind of a platform with springs, and they will load this thing up with wood and they can go off and leave it but it's going to keep fighting. Sometimes when I get up and feel the blood sugar is high, I will envision them coming down into the streams and chipping away some of the pollution that has gotten in there. Then they will load this up and carry it back and put it into the steam engine.

Researcher: You do this generally when you are running or feeling bad in the morning?

Dave: I try to do this all during the day. I will try to think about it.

Researcher: Kind of a positive image to replace the worry that you have?

Dave: Yes, I always think about it when I run. Always. I try to think about it during the day too. Not as intensely as I do when I run because my running can last anywhere from 30 minutes to an hour and that is a very private time for me. I don't want anyone screwing with me and I can think about this. I really concentrate.

Researcher: I am curious why would you just restrict it to two people? Why not bring in a group or a militia or army?

Dave: It just seemed like two people could do it. I guess that it's just a testimony of strength too. It's a personal battle and I figure if this man is strong enough with some help from the woman he will do it and I can do it too. It takes a lot of work to do this thinking and you can get burned out on it so what I do sometimes is this. I will have them build a giant pile of wood and say they are going on vacation 3-4 days but they know they have got enough wood to last till they get back.

Researcher: That is a very usual thing to do, many patients do this. It takes a lot of energy to continue to focus thinking, as you said.

Dave: One thing I have added since I even talked to you is a woman having this beautiful orchard and fruit trees and she has dug a channel over there herself. The man has helped her some but it is mainly her work and she is growing this tremendous fruit and she will let water go over there and will get this basket of fruit full of giant, luscious fruit; nectarines and grapes, I can almost taste them when I think about it. This piece of land is really my pancreas, growing this great fruit which means it is really working. You see a lot of baskets of grapes.

Researcher: The steam engine itself, is it pumping water?

Dave: Yes, it's pumping water. It's helping to build up and it's going to go down into the body, it is actually the pancreas. Also, I have used this sometimes to think of the steam engine in terms of my heart pumping blood. Also, I have been reading all of this junk about kidneys and I really got worried about it. So one day when I was running I just decided that the man and woman should go inside this big wooden room, this giant room. There's a kind of a pit you know, a well with rocks. It's an old well you know, not a very pleasant place and they just decide, "Well, we are going to cap this thing and shut it up and never look at it again. And we are going to build this huge wooden covering over this well on which they chop down trees and whatever." I have not had any back pains since they capped the well.

160

Researcher: Do you have any notion or idea of what your imagery is actually doing to your body from a physical standpoint?

Dave: I don't know, but I have my own thoughts. I think sometimes you only feel bad because somebody else says you should. What I think I am making my mind do to my body is really making me aware of how healthy I am.

Researcher: Then what you are doing is keeping in touch with your body?

Dave: Yes. I get to thinking about my grandfather who lived till he was 96 years old on my father's side and I feel that if I have that blood in me and the man lived till he was 96 and died of a natural death I have got a lot going for me.

Researcher: Didn't you tell us you were the only one in your family with diabetes?

Dave: Right, as far as I know. I found a first cousin who has it now but for years I was the only one in my family.

Researcher: What has been your physician's response to your rather outstanding physical condition?

Dave: He says I must be taking care of myself. Also, I wanted to tell you this, all diabetics take shots, either in the side, stomach, or arms. I take mine in my thighs and stomach. As a result of constant shooting up you develop what they call insulin knots which is just really your fault, you have not rotated the needle enough and it causes a knot to form. A tumor is what it looks like. I had one in my left thigh for nearly 2 years and last year I went to the doctor and he said, "Well, rest the thigh a little bit," so I would rest it and that thing still had not gone away and even when I talked to you a few months ago it had not gone away. So 2 weeks ago I started this thing. What I did was have the woman in my imagery dig a stream down in the valley. There is a big rock and she wants to get rid of it and so she starts beating at the thing with a hoe and building a bigger opening to her dam and she will let the water rush in, eat away, and the water is rushing by. The more water, the more it will work away this piece of rock. And do you know that thing was gone in about 2 weeks?

161

OBESITY

About one of every five people is fat enough to be called in a general way "obese." Some authorities place the incidence of obesity at 25% of the population. Obesity, depending on its extent, causes a wide variety of damage. Metropolitan Life Insurance Company statistics have shown that for a man of 45 an increase of 25 pounds above standard weight cuts life expectancy by 25%. Obesity may contribute to cardiac failure due to the extra load in increased need for circulation. Osteoarthritis often is related to the extra weight on the joints, as well as atherosclerosis.

Although there are numerous diseases associated with obesity, treatment of obesity is unsuccessful in most cases. Follow-up studies of patients after one year generally find that most patients gained back what they had lost. In fact, the cure rate for obesity is said to be not much better than for cancer.

In a recent interview with a director of Diet Workshop, "A Motivational Dimension in Weight Reduction," the concept of imagery was related to their focus for achievement. The director was enthusiastic about her successes and could articulate the positive outcome of weight control for several of her cases. The conclusion to the discussion was that a measure of imagery for obesity was important for diagnostic and intervention purposes.

The following dialogue is a part of that interview (D representing director and R for researcher):

D: First, let me tell you a little of my history. I was grossly obese all my life. But as I was losing my weight, I had a hard time overcoming the loss because in my mind I could hear my mother telling me to keep my strength up. I had a doctor who kept convincing me to lose weight because he said, "You will find you will have more energy." I knew what he was saying was correct, but what mother teaches you at home stays with you, and this is what all of our teaching in the workshop is really about. You can overcome that and say, "Okay, now I'm an adult."

R: Could you, looking back, now give us an idea of what was going on in your body?

D: No, because I wasn't medically trained to what was going on in my body. More so with my mind. But with the body I had no idea. Only when I lost the weight was I able to accept what happened within the body. What we're finding is if someone has never dieted before, they can lose weight beautifully, because they simply follow the directions. But if somebody has tried it, then you have a combination of things. Again it's with "mind programming" I'm sure, because they feel that they already know it and so they don't really have to practice it.

R: Did you picture yourself thin?

D: Yes.

R: How did you do that?

D: I had pictures. You know, I came from a poor family, but I had catalog pictures and I would look at something and think, "Now I would like to look like that." This is the way that we proceed with our clients, rather than emphasizing the nutritional and medical aspects of overweight.

R: How do you help your clients image themselves thin?

D: We do it through classroom work. It's very much along the mind control bit. We ask, "Can you picture yourself thinner?" and we keep stressing it each time they attend. We'll do something like we may ask, "How much weight do you think you can lose?" We do contests along that line. I'll tell you of an experiment that I did. I had a class of 149 members and just for an experiment, on my own, I decided that I was going to try something to see how members see themselves. As the members came in through the door I gave them a slip of paper and asked them to put down whether they expected to lose over the upcoming Christmas holiday or whether they expected to gain weight. I only wanted a "+" or "−." They put this down and they kept it with them. The other thing I asked them to do was not weigh at home, to trust me and that I would be the only one to weigh them. I didn't want them to monitor their progress on the scales. The following week they came in, and out of 149 people only five guessed incorrectly. One guessed wrong because in her mind she decided she was going to have a piece of cake with family that was coming in, and she put down a plus. She had lost because one piece of cake will not permit you to gain weight. But a total of five guessed incorrectly out of 149 people and I was just fascinated because of their accuracy.

So, as with the findings on cancer, people with weight problems are able to predict quite accurately their future bodily condition, at least in the short run. They seem to have insight into behaviors that involve weight gain, and thus a handle on weight control that few obese people are willing to acknowledge. And secondly, interdigitated into the process is the notion of imagery: picturing in the mind's eye the size and shape desired, and learning to respond in accordance with a new self-image.

THE COMMON COLD

The "common" cold has traditionally been the disease of which we are most aware. Very few escape at least one bout per year with the symptoms of a runny nose, froggy throat, and achy feelings. The "cold" is not one disease, but a variety of diseases that affect similar membranes and manifest similar symptoms. Nevertheless, the maladies usually infect the majority of the population, especially the school children, and it is common knowledge that some students are more prone to colds than others. Little research has been done in the area on personality factors that correlate to absenteeism in schools, but it is likely to be similar to the factors in adult absenteeism in industry.

In an effort to develop some pilot work to see what imagery differences exist between high- and low-absenteeism students, a 7th-grade class and a 9th-grade class from Levelland Junior High School, Levelland, Texas[1], were asked to draw images of their disease process when they had a cold.

[1]Appreciation for the coordination of data collection is given to Mary Lou Lawlis, Director of Guidance, Levelland, Texas.

They listened to a tape that included a programmed fantasy trip through their bodies and a brief explanation of the mechanisms of immunological defenses. After the total class listened to the complete tape, they were asked to draw the way they saw their bodies defend against colds in whatever manner they wished. Those students whose absentee record was greater than 25% over the last 60-day quarter were compared to those students who had less than 5% absentee rates due to reasons of illness.

The obvious result is that students can and do use imagery in some form when they consider illness. All but one of the forty were able to draw some representation that could be understood as dynamic process. More importantly, they were all different in the sense that virtually every picture was drawn in a unique fashion featuring various levels of conceptualization, figures, methods of figure interaction, and artistic abilities. This result reflects the fact that the students were not programmed or instructed to perform their tasks in any specific manner.

The tasks of the evaluator were to study the commonalities in this low-absentee group and compare them with the high-absentee group. The drawings are quite different in quality. The most striking difference between the two groups was the amount of space occupied by the drawings. For example, three of the six high-attendance drawings covered most of the page, and the remainder of the group's drawings covered at least 25% of the page. None of the high-absentee group drawings covered more than 25% of the page.

The high-attendance group's drawings were also much more fantasized, with two representing more than one stage of process. Only one of the high-absentee group had action figures, and his appeared to relate to a more personal message such as a parental relationship between a father and son, rather than activities within his body.

These findings are related to the dimensions of consistency and vividness, and pertain to the individual's investment in the process as pictorially presented. Drawings that are low on these dimensions usually reflect individuals who are either too far removed from understanding their body, unable to relate to their feelings about their body, or too overwhelmed or frightened to consider their own participation in the disease process.

Another interesting difference was that in the low-absentee group's pictures there was an obvious "good guy" and "bad guy." Again, the moralistic component possesses some emotional and righteous energy that might be related to the investment to remaining well (Dimension 8). For example, it was noted that at least 50% of all the drawings contained a representation of a devil. It may have been the philosophy of some of the students' religion that disease was a retribution for sin or a test of faith (as in the case of Job), however, information on religious backgrounds was not available.

Thus, this study indicates that students can use imagery to represent their body's defenses. Size, consistency, and moralistic projection appeared to differ in the two extreme groups with regard to absentee records.

The implications of this research are far reaching for the public school. For example, if a teacher knew which students would be most susceptible to colds, a more flexible curriculum might be envisioned or perhaps teacher selection which would be more compatible to the more absentee-prone students might be considered.

ANGELS AND CROWNS

The cancer patients that we studied would frequently report a very profound spontaneous imagery experience involving visualizations of religious figures. The "visits" were very much a source of comfort to the patients, with visions of another existence offering a particular sustenance to them as they approached death. Several patients reported pre-diagnostic information, which included tumor placements and descriptions, as well as more positive information regarding prognosis of return to health. We were not studying this type of imagery systematically, and any verification of the pre-diagnostic information had to be based on the patient's verbalization combined with whatever we could glean from medical records. Suffice to say, though, we could find no contradictory evidence using these two sources of information.

Our pilot efforts to study this intriguing phenomena began with the serendipitous finding by Ms. Harriett Gibbs, our researcher, that exactly half of the patients interviewed by her over a 3-week period *volunteered* information on spiritual visualizations. All of the patients interviewed were designated by members of the rehabilitation team to be the most imminently close to death of the patients being treated. Our study of them, which was subsumed under a project evaluation effort, dealt primarily with death anxiety and religious values, with the goal being to better understand and to more carefully meet the needs of the dying patients of lower socioeconomic levels—a sadly neglected group in the thanatological literature. The patients were tested with Templer's Death Anxiety Scale (Templer, 1970), Allport's Religious Orientation Scale (Allport & Ross, 1967), and interviewed, using a structured format. It was in conjunction with the latter that information was volunteered about the spiritual visions.

The dialogue that follows represents excerpts from an interview with a 53-year-old woman with widely metastatic breast cancer (R = researcher, P = patient):

R: When you pray for strength, what kind of strength is it that you pray for?

P: It's just that God give me strength, and help me to do the things that I want to do. And it comes, the strength. When I was in the hospital—getting back to that—after I'd passed out and stayed out a couple of days, I woke up upstairs, and I commenced to try to move my arms and legs and I couldn't move them. And I come to and I looked around the room and I said where in the Lord am I at. That's the first thing that popped into my mind. And the next morning I said God give me strength. And you know that I felt strength going from my head down to my toes. I felt it, and it came everyday.

R: That must have been quite a feeling.

P: It was, and I'll tell you something else. Christ came and sat down on my bed and talked to me.

167

R: What was that like? Tell me about that.

P: It was beautiful. I told the doctor the day before, I've got something wrong with my head. I said I've got tumors or something in my head. He said, Oh no you don't. So that night I said, God, tell me please what's wrong with me. I've got to know or I'll go crazy. Well that night I laid there and I prayed that night for him to tell me what it was and he told me exactly how many tumors I had in my head. I had seven. So the next morning when the doctor came up there, I said, doctor, I have got cancers of the brain. I said I've got eight of them up there, little bitty uns—they're here.

R: What did he say to that?

P: He said, Oh no, not a chance. I said I'll lay you odds, I bet you your next five years' salary that I've got tumors of the brain. He said, Nah. You know too much—you're too smart now to have tumors of the brain. I said maybe so but I says it's not me; I didn't say I had 'em, God told me I had 'em. Believe you me boy, you better believe me. 'Cause I said Christ knows everything.

R: When Christ came and sat down on your bed and told you you had brain tumors did you see anything?

P: I saw him sitting on the foot of the bed. He was sitting and he had a purple robe on and there was a halo of light around his head but I never did completely see the full of his face, just the side, it was a profile.

R: Was it a scary thing?

P: No.

R: How did you know who it was?

P: I just knew because I was living so close to God.

R: Did he talk to you or did you just know what he was saying?

P: I didn't hear a word He said but I either dreamt it or He told me. It had to be. Because I saw his vision there on the foot of the bed and I visioned I heard his voice. If he hadn't told me I had tumors up here how would I have known it? All my trouble started right here in the back of the neck.

After that I said take me to brain scan, all right, they did. They showed up, seven of them.

R: What did the doctor say to you, didn't he wonder again how you knew?

P: Well I told him I knew! I said Christ told me. I don't care whether he believed me or not.

R: Do you think he believed you?

P: No, I don't think he did. Because he's one of those skeptical guys—you have to knock 'em dead with it.

Our attempts to verify the patient's information have been successful only to the extent that a bone scan taken after the admission in question does show a brain mass. Nevertheless, there is no question that the patient is comforted and strengthened by her experience.

The next dialogue is of another sort; it was offered by a college-educated, 28-year-old male who had a "death" experience during surgery with very vivid recollection of the images involved:

P: There was something I was going to tell you that you may not want to hear at all, and may be off the subject but I had a real experience, I almost died.

R: Can you describe that for me?

P: Well I remember I was in a lot of pain and was real sick and then all of a sudden it was like the hospital room was right there getting smaller and smaller and I was in a tunnel and then I was in this garden, really beautiful colors like apricots and taupes, and those colors, just real soothing and there were these beings floating, and it was my totality, my body was there, it wasn't like a dream. It was a different body because it did not hurt and I was in control of everything whereas I had not been and there was this beautiful garden and we just walked through it and all of a sudden way back in the tunnel I heard the nurse saying, "Wake up and I said no I really can't, I need to stay here, this is really fine. Enjoying this. It's like the voices sort of drew me back and I woke up and was in the hospital room.

R: When you had that experience, were you talking with anybody that was there in that place? Were you able to communicate with anybody there?

169

P: Not in words, but it was like communication but a non-verbal thing, through ESP. I had never read Kubler-Ross or anything like that before this. Then I read some of that stuff—and there was this river, but I never crossed the river, which is real typical of this type of experience I understand. We communicated though because I remember asking lots of questions. They were really transferring answers to me. It was almost a sacred thing, not something you talk about.

His "death" experience has quite naturally influenced his conception of an after-life.

R: When you think of your own death, what do you see as happening?

P: At the point of death, there will be a total cessation of pain, a real release. There won't be any unfamiliarity, a total sense of belonging. Every imagineable color, just brilliant. I feel like if heaven is even 1/10 of what I've been told all my life, then that's fine with me. The Christian experience, if it's going to deliver even a portion, that's fine with me. And to me the excitement is finally having all the answers and being in what I call communion with your source.

R: What's going to take you on this journey? What will you be like? Are you going to go back through the tunnel?

P: My soul will leave my body and I will see that, that will be a very real thing to me. I'll have heavenly spirits that will accompany me on my journey. I think it'll be a journey, maybe through a tunnel, definitely to another dimension. After that there won't be a need for guides. It'll be a familiar situation. That's because the more you're familiar with God the better able you'll be to relate to him when you're finally there in his presence. I think you'll know who it is. It's a utopia. There are times when I really feel a real heavy spiritual presence. It's always in the nick of time.

In retrospect, we examined the data we had collected on the patients interviewed to determine whether the group who spontaneously expressed the visualizations were different from the other patients in any way. Indeed, there was a pronounced tendency for the patients who admitted the

visions to score "intrinsic" on Allport's Scale. In his description of religious types, he identified four basic orientations:
intrinsic, extrinsic, indiscriminately pro- and indiscriminately
anti-religious. Intrinsic people generally find a master motive
in religion; for them it is a livable dogma in that they seek to
live the teachings of their faith. In other words, their religious
beliefs are well integrated into their lives. Extrinsic scorers,
on the other hand, are more self-centered, more likely to use
their religion in a utilitarian fashion or with an eye toward
what it can do for them. Protection from Hell, for instance,
would be an extrinsic use of religion. The indiscriminately pro-
religious scorer would have a tendency to agree with *all* the
religious statements, while the indiscriminately anti-religious
would disagree with all religious statements. The patients
who did not report visualizations were a mixture of all four
types (but primarily extrinsically religious). The individuals
who reported visions also had slightly lower death anxiety
scores than did the nonreporting group.

    These studies are not being included because of the
statistical significance of the results, but rather because they
seem to relate—in a yet undefinable fashion—to the research
on cancer imagery. In both cases—the spiritual visions and in
the images of cancer—we are encountering unconscious
material which is part of the patients' reality. Whether it is
part of our reality or not is relatively unimportant, for it
deserves attention as a major behavioral determinant.

REFERENCES

Achterberg, J., Lawlis, G. F., Simonton, O. C., & Simonton, S. Psychological factors and blood chemistries as disease outcome predictors for cancer patients. *Multivariate Clinical Experimental Research*, December, 1977.

Achterberg, J., Simonton, O. C., & Matthews-Simonton, S. *Stress, psychological factors and cancer: An annotated bibliography.* Fort Worth: New Medicine Press, 1976.

Allport, G., & Ross, J. Personal religious orientation and prejudice. *Journal of Personality and Social Psychology*, 1967, *5*, 432-443.

Bacon, C. L., Renneker, R., & Cutler, M. A psychosomatic survey of cancer of the breast. *Psychosomatic Medicine*, 1952, *14*, 543.

Bahnson, C. B., & Bahnson, M. B. Cancer as an alternative to psychosis: A theoretical model for somatic and psychologic regression. In D. M. Kissen & L. LeShan (Eds), *Psychosomatic aspects of neoplastic disease*. Philadelphia: Lippincott, 1964, 184. (a)

Bahnson, C. B., & Bahnson, M. B. Denial and repression of primitive impulses and of disturbing emotions in patients with malignant neoplasms. In D. M. Kissen & L. LeShan (Eds), *Psychosomatic aspects of neoplastic disease*. Philadelphia: Lippincott, 1964, 42. (b)

Bahnson, C. B., & Bahnson, M. B. Role of the ego defenses: Denial and repression in the etiology of malignant neoplasm. In E. M. Weyer (Ed.), *Annals of the New York Academy of Sciences*, 1966, *125*(3), 827.

Benson, H. *The relaxation response.* New York: William Morrow, 1975.

Betts, G. H. *The distribution and functions of mental imagery.* Teachers College: Contributions to Education, 1909.

Blumberg, E. M. Results of psychological testing of cancer patients. In J. A. Gengerelli & F. J. Kirkner (Eds), *The psychological variables in human cancer*. Berkeley: University of California Press, 1954, 30.

173

Booth, G. Cancer and humanism. In D. M. Kissen & L. LeShan (Eds), *Psychosomatic aspects of neoplastic disease.* Philadelphia: Lippincott, 1964, 159.

Brown, B. *New mind, new body.* New York: Harper & Row, 1974.

Bugental, J. F. T. Discussion of E. M. Blumberg's article, Results of psychological testing of cancer patients. In J. A. Gengerelli & F. J. Kirkner (Eds), *The psychological variables in human cancer.* Berkeley: University of California Press, 1954, 95.

Cautela, J. The use of covert conditioning in hypnotherapy. *International Journal of Clinical and Experimental Hypnosis*, 1975, *23*, 15.

Cobb, Beatrix. A socio-psychological study of the cancer patient. Unpublished doctoral dissertation, University of Texas, Austin, 1952.

Coppen, A. J., & Metcalfe, M. Cancer and extraversion. In D. M. Kissen & L. LeShan (Eds), *Psychosomatic aspects of neoplastic disease.* Philadelphia: Lippincott, 1964.

Darwin, C. R. *The origin of the species by means of natural selection, or, the preservation of favored races in the struggle for life* (6th ed.). London: John Murray, 1901.

Ellis, F. W., & Blumberg, E. M. Comparative case summaries with psychological profiles in representative rapidly and slowly progressive neoplastic diseases. In J. A. Gengerelli & F. J. Kirkner (Eds), *The psychological variables in human cancer.* Berkeley: University of California Press, 1954, 72.

Evans, E. *A psychological study of cancer.* New York: Dodd, Mead, 1926.

Evans, R. B., Stern, E., & Marmorston, J. Psychological-hormonal relationships in men with cancer. *Psychological Reports*, 1965, *17*, 715.

Foque, E. Le probleme du cancer dans ses aspects psychiques. *Gaz. Hop. Paris*, 1931, *104*, 827.

Fowler, J. E., Budzynski, T. H., & Vandenbergh, R. L. Effects of an EMG biofeedback relaxation program on the control of diabetes: A case study. *Biofeedback and Self-Regulation*, 1976, *1*, 1.

Greene, W. A. Psychological factors in reticuloendothelial disease. *Psychosomatic Medicine*, 1954, *16*, 220.

Greene, W. A. The psychosocial setting of the development of leukemia and lymphoma. In E. M. Weyer (Ed.), *Annals of the New York Academy of Sciences*, 1966, *125*(3), 794.

174

Greene, W. A., Young, L., & Swisher, S. M. Psychological factors and reticuloendothelial disease. II. Observations on a group of women with lymphomas and leukemias. *Psychosomatic Medicine*, 1956, *18*, 284.

Hathaway, S. R., & McKinley, J. C. *Minnesota multiphasic personality inventory*. New York: Psychological Corporation, 1943.

Hinkle, L. E., Christenson, W., Benjamin, B., & Wolf, H. G. Observations on the role of nasal adaptive reactions, emotions and life situations in the genesis of minor respiratory illnesses. *Psychosomatic Medicine*, 1962, *24*, 515.

Holt, R. R. Imagery: The return of the ostracized. *American Psychologist*, 1964, *19*, 254-264.

Huckabee, M. Introversion-extroversion and imagery. *Psychological Reports*, 1974, *34*, 453-454.

Inman, O. B. Development of two different types of cancer in a patient undergoing psychoanalytic treatment. In D. M. Kissen & L. LeShan (Eds), *Psychosomatic aspects of neoplastic disease*. Philadelphia: Lippincott, 1964.

Izsak, F. C., & Medalie, J. H. Comprehensive follow-up of carcinoma patients. *Journal of Chronic Disease*, 1971, *24*, 179-191.

Jacobs, J. S. L. Cancer: Host-resistance and host-acquiescence. In J. A. Gengerelli & F. J. Kirkner (Eds), *The psychological variables in human cancer*. Berkeley: University of California Press, 1954, 128.

Jacobsen, E. *Progressive relaxation*. Chicago: University of Chicago Press, 1942.

Jung, C. G. *Psychology and alchemy*. Princeton, N.J.: Princeton University Press, 1968.

Khatina, J. Vividness of imagery and creative self-perception. *The Gifted Child Quarterly*, 1975, *19*(1), 33-37.

Kissen, D. M. The significance of personality in lung cancer in men. In E. M. Weyer (Ed.), *Annals of the New York Academy of Sciences*, 1966, *125*(3), 820.

Kissen, D. M. Psychosocial factors, personality and lung cancer in men aged 55-64. *British Journal of Medical Psychology*, 1967, *40*, 29.

Kissen, D. M., & Eysenck, H. J. Personality in male lung cancer patients. *Journal of Psychosomatic Research*, 1962, *6*, 123.

175

Klopfer, B. Psychological variables in human cancer. *Journal of Projective Techniques*, 1957, *21*, 331-340.

Koenig, R., Levin, S. M., & Brennan, M. J. The emotional status of cancer patients as measured by a psychological test. *Journal of Chronic Disability*, 1967, *20*, 923.

Lamarck, J. *Philosophie zoologique*. Paris: J. B. Balliere, 1830.

Lawlis, G. F., & Lu, E. Judgment of counseling process: Reliability, agreement and error. *Psychological Bulletin*, 1972, *78*, 17-20.

LeShan, L. An emotional life history pattern associated with neoplastic disease. In E. M. Weyer (Ed.), *Annals of the New York Academy of Sciences*, 1966, *125*, 3.

LeShan, L., & Worthington, R. E. Some recurrent life-history patterns observed in patients with malignant disease. *Journal of Nervous and Mental Disease*, 1956, *124*, 460.

Levenson, H. Distinctions within the concept of internal-external control: Development of a new scale. *Proceedings of the American Psychological Association*, 1972, 259-260.

Luria, A. *The mind of a mnemonist*. New York: Basic Books, 1968.

Luthe, W. *Autogenic therapy*. Vol. I-VI. New York: Grune & Stratton, 1969.

Miller, R. F., & Jones, H. W. The possibility of precipitating the leukemia state by emotional factors. *Blood*, 1948, *8*, 880.

Muslin, H. L., Gyarfas, K., & Pieper, W. J. Separation experience and cancer of the breast. In E. M. Weyer (Ed.), *Annals of the New York Academy of Sciences*, 1966, *125*(3), 802.

Neisser, V. The processes of vision. In A. Richardson (Ed.) *Perception, mechanism and models*. San Francisco: Freeman, 1972.

Nemeth, G., & Mezei, A. Personality traits of cancer patients compared with benign tumor patients on the basis of the Rorschach test. In D. M. Kissen and L. LeShan (Eds), *Psychosomatic aspects of neoplastic disease*. Philadelphia: Lippincott, 1954, 12.

Netzer, M. The body image of women under study for cancer. Unpublished dissertation, Yeshiva University, New York, 1965.

Paget, I. *Surgical pathology*. (2nd ed.) London: Longmons, 1870.

Palmer, R. D., & Field, P. B. Visual imagery and susceptibility to hypnosis. *Journal of Consulting and Clinical Psychology*, 1968, *32*, 456-461.

Paloucek, F. P., & Graham, J. B. The influence of psychosocial factors on the prognosis in cancer of the cervix. In E. M. Weyer (Ed.), *Annals of the New York Academy of Sciences*, 1966, *125*(3), 814.

Paivio, A. Mental imagery in associative learning and memory. *Psychological Review*, 1969, *76*, 241-263.

Pelletier, K. R. *Mind as healer, mind as slayer.* New York: Dell, 1977.

Prehn, R. T. The relationship of immunology to carcinogenesis. *Annals of the New York Academy of Science*, 1969, *164*, 449-459.

Reznikoff, M. Psychological factors in breast cancer. *Psychosomatic Medicine*, 1955, *17*, 96.

Richardson, A. *Mental imagery.* London: Routledge & Kegan Paul, 1969.

Riley, V. Mouse mammary tumors: Alteration of incidence as apparent function of stress. *Science*, 1975, *189*, 465-467.

Samuels, M., & Samuels, N. *Seeing with the mind's eye.* New York and Berkeley: Random House, 1975.

Schutz, W. C. *The FIRO-B scales: Manual.* Palo Alto, Calif.: Consulting Psychologists Press, 1967.

Selye, H. *The stress of life.* New York: McGraw-Hill, 1956.

Sheehan, P. Stimulus imagery effect and the role of imagery in incidental learning. *Australian Journal of Psychology*, 1973, *25*, 93-102.

Simonton, O. C., & Simonton, S. Belief systems and the management of the emotional aspects of malignancy. *Journal of Transpersonal Psychology*, 1975, *7*, 29-47.

Snow, H. L. *Clinical notes on cancer.* London: Churchill, 1883.

Snow, H. L. *The reappearance of cancer after apparent extirpation.* London: Churchill, 1890.

Snow, H. L. *Cancer and the cancer process.* London: Churchill, 1893.

Solomon, G. F., & Amkraut, A. A. Emotions, stress, and immunity. *Frontiers of Radiation Therapeutic Oncology*, 1972, *1*, 84-96.

177

Tarlau, M., & Smalheiser, I. Personality patterns in patients with malignant tumors of the breast and cervix: An exploratory study. *Psychosomatic Medicine*, 1951, *13*, 117.

Templer, D. The construction and validation of a death anxiety scale. *The Journal of General Psychology*, 1970, *82*, 165-177.

Thomas, C. B. Precursors of premature disease and death. *Annals of Internal Medicine*, 1976, *85*, 653-658.

Wagman, R., & Stewart, C. Visual imagery and hypnotic susceptibility. *Perceptual and Motor Skills*, 1974, *38*, 815-822.

Walshe, W. A. *The nature and treatment of cancer.* London: Taylor and Walton, 1846.

Wheeler, J. P., & Caldwell, B. McD. Psychological evaluation of women with cancer of the breast and of the cervix. *Psychosomatic Medicine*, 1955, *17*, 256.

AUTHOR INDEX

SUBJECT INDEX

About the Authors

Jeanne Achterberg received a Ph.D. in 1973 from Texas Christian University, with a major course of study in physiological psychology. Using a combination of her knowledge in physiology, psychodiagnostics, and research design and analysis, she developed the initial research program for the Cancer Counseling and Research Center in Ft. Worth. She has consulted with numerous private clinics, state agencies, and institutions on the management and development of research programs on the psychological aspects of cancer, and is a frequent lecturer on the topic. She was co-director of an evaluation team for a Cancer Demonstration Project at the University of Texas Health Science Center, Dallas, where she currently holds the academic rank of Assistant Professor of Physical Medicine. She and Dr. Lawlis developed the PERCEPT concept—a series of materials designed for patient education, and is one of the founders of Consultants for Patient and Physican Communication (CPPC). She is continuing her research in an area newly and broadly defined as Behavioral Medicine—identifying psychological components of the course of disease and implementing appropriate behavioral treatment methodology for a variety of disorders including arthritis, diabetes, trauma, as well as cancer.

G. Frank Lawlis received his Ph.D. in psychology in 1968 from Texas Tech University with specialization in Rehabilitation, after completing an intensive internship at New York University Medical Center. After serving as Director of Research at University of Arkansas Rehabilitation Research Center, he returned to Texas Tech and served as Director of Rehabilitation Psychology from 1970 to 1975. Dr. Lawlis has also worked at Audie Murphy VA Hospital, as Acting Chief of Psychology and Associate Professor of Psychiatry at the University of Texas Health Center in San Antonio. He is currently Associate Professor of Psychology at North Texas State University and Associate Professor of Physical Medicine at the University of Texas Health Science Center at Dallas. Having a Diplomate in Counseling Psychology and writing several articles in statistical methodology, including a book, *Multivariate Techniques for the Behavioral Scientist*, has helped facilitate his research and clinical pursuits in such fields as conjoint psychological methods to disease intervention and pain, program evaluation, group and family counseling, bioenergetics, and vocational behavior.